"Steve Larson's n
offers readers the
a world that often ᴜᴜɢᴍᴀᴛɪᴢᴇs those who struggle with mental
health issues."

Mark Batterson, *New York Times* bestselling author,
The Circle Maker

"*The Four Keys to Mental Health* is a timely and Spirit-led guide
for anyone navigating emotional and mental challenges. With biblical wisdom and practical insight, Steve offers hope, healing, and
a clear path forward. I believe this book will equip the church to
care for hearts and minds in a powerful new way."

Rob Ketterling, lead pastor, River Valley Church

"The Bible places a high value on mental health. It shows the
interconnectedness of the spirit, soul, and body, advocating for
holistic health. Steve Larson uses Scripture and biblical principles
to take you on a journey to experience higher levels of mental and
spiritual well-being in Christ!"

Doug Clay, general superintendent, Assemblies of God, USA;
vice chairman, World Assemblies of God Fellowship

"The content that Pastor Steve Larson presents in *The Four Keys
to Mental Health* has been honed over a lifetime of effective ministry. His transparency is refreshing, relevant, and powerful. The
wealth of information he shares stems from personal experience
and the Scriptures. I highly recommend you invest the time to read
this enlightening work."

Mark Dean, superintendent, Minnesota District
of the Assemblies of God

"One of the greatest challenges leaders face today is the quiet drift
from joy—a mysterious emptiness that replaces the passion they
once had for their calling. If you've found yourself in that place,
The Four Keys to Mental Health offers a timely and practical
guide. With clarity and compassion, Steve Larson delivers simple

yet powerful strategies to help you reclaim the joy, purpose, and mental wellness needed to thrive in what you love to do."

Dr. Douglas M. Graham, assistant superintendent,
Minnesota District of the Assemblies of God;
former interim president, North Central University

"Steve Larson first caught my attention when he planted a church in a small town in southeastern Minnesota. I watched and cheered from the sidelines as that church grew and began to thrive under his capable leadership and then found myself, along with several others, walking alongside him as he struggled through a period of deep depression. We all celebrated with him as he worked his way through to a place of health and an even greater place of strength and influence. Steve has used the insights and lessons learned from this difficult period in his life to help and encourage countless numbers of pastors and Christian leaders. His message on this topic has been so impactful that our Minnesota ministry network uses him to share his story with our entry-level ministerial candidates each year at our credentialing seminar. I highly recommend *The Four Keys to Mental Health* as a personal help or resource for any leader."

Clarence St. John, former superintendent,
Minnesota District of the Assemblies of God

"Many people at some point in their lives find themselves experiencing an inner conflict between 'How I think I should be' and 'How I truly am.' Steve Larson skillfully weaves parts of his own story into a comprehensive collection of truths, wisdom, and insight for anyone, especially Christians and ministers, who struggle with this conflict. This book will encourage, educate, and hopefully inspire you to take the steps necessary for greater personal and relational health."

Tim Ruden, MDiv, PhD, LPCC

The Four Keys to Mental Health

The Four Keys to Mental Health

HOW TO FEEL BETTER, THINK CLEARLY, AND ENJOY LIFE AGAIN

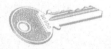

STEVE LARSON

Chosen

a division of Baker Publishing Group
Minneapolis, Minnesota

Published by Chosen Books
Minneapolis, Minnesota
ChosenBooks.com

Chosen Books is a division of
Baker Publishing Group, Grand Rapids, Michigan

Printed in the United States of America

Library of Congress Cataloging-in-Publication Data
Names: Larson, Steve author
Title: The four keys to mental health : how to feel better, think clearly, and enjoy life again / Steve Larson.
Description: Minneapolis, Minnesota : Chosen, a division of Baker Publishing Group, [2026] | Includes bibliographical references.
Identifiers: LCCN 2025016501 | ISBN 9780800773243 paperback | ISBN 9780800778439 casebound | ISBN 9781493452941 ebook
Subjects: LCSH: Mental health—Religious aspects—Christianity
Classification: LCC BT732.4 .L386 2026 | DDC 261.8/322—dc23/eng/20250825
LC record available at https://lccn.loc.gov/2025016501

This publication is intended to provide helpful and informative material on the subjects addressed. Readers should consult their personal health professionals before adopting any of the suggestions in this book or drawing inferences from it. The author and publisher expressly disclaim responsibility for any adverse effects arising from the use or application of the information contained in this book.

Cover design by Chris Kuhatschek

Author is represented by the literary agency of The Blythe Daniel Agency, Inc.

Baker Publishing Group publications use paper produced from sustainable forestry practices and postconsumer waste whenever possible.

26 27 28 29 30 31 32   7 6 5 4 3 2 1

To Tammy, Dalton, and Miracle—
because of you, I am a "famillionaire."

Contents

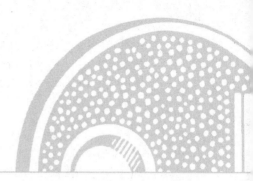

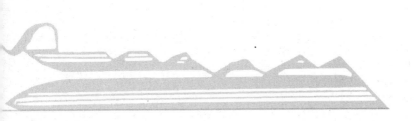

Foreword

Pastor Steve Larson has written a book for both mental health professionals and pastors who work with individuals struggling with mental health challenges. He presents evidence-based mental health strategies in an easy-to-read format incorporating relevant Scripture passages that are meaningful and often challenging. Drawing from personal experiences and biblical examples, Larson connects deeply with readers who are struggling.

Pastor Larson's honest account of his own journey with depression —including the recurrence, loneliness, denial, and shame—will resonate with many, particularly Christians who feel isolated in their suffering. For pastors who have not personally experienced depression, this book offers insight into the anguish many congregants face. Larson emphasizes God's presence in suffering and His desire for individuals to grow in His values and virtues amid pain. He supports this with key Scripture passages that affirm God's love and compassion.

Throughout the book, Pastor Larson weaves in practical pychological concepts from cognitive behavioral therapy, acceptance and commitment therapy, and dialectical behavioral therapy. These approaches help readers manage negative thinking and emotional distress. Medical professionals will also appreciate Larson's emphasis on lifestyle fundamentals—exercise, nutrition, sleep, leisure, and balance. His reflection on relationship challenges integrated with personal experiences and biblical wisdom adds depth. Larson approaches the topic of psychiatric medication with balance and nuance. He encourages thoughtful consideration, helping readers weigh the decision within a holistic framework.

Each chapter concludes with daily reflections, Scriptures to memorize, and journaling prompts—tools designed to address negative thoughts and encourage spititual growth. Larson also provides guidance on managing nighttime rumination, ending each chapter with a prayer focused on God's presence, faithfulness, and care.

The book concludes with a Checklist of Care, summarizing each chapter's key points. This summary serves as a call to action from anxious and depressive pitfalls toward committed values and relationships. This book will become a frequently used resource among Christian counselors and pastors.

Thank you, Pastor Larson, for your vulnerability, and for sharing the lessons that God has taught you and your family on this continued personal journey. May God bless your obedience in writing this book.

Jeanne M. Allen,
PsyD, LP, APRN, CNS

The Gains of the Gathering Years

Darkness is my closest friend.

Psalm 88:18

What's there to be happy about? That thought passed through my mind while waiting for my doctor's appointment. The nurses instructed me to fill out a form on depression:

- Do you have a loss of interest in usual things? *Yes.*
- Do you have feelings of hopelessness and worthlessness? *Yes.*
- Have you gained weight or lost weight? *Yes, I lost twenty pounds. I was so anxious that I didn't want to eat.*
- Do you have sleep disturbances? *Yes, I was constantly fatigued and had difficulty getting out of bed in the morning.*

As I filled it out, I felt hopeless. I looked at the people sitting in the waiting room and felt so dark on the inside that it was as if I was wearing tinted glasses. Everything seemed bleak. It felt

13

as though the light had gone out in my life. I could relate to the people I had heard say, "I have so much sorrow that I don't know if I can face tomorrow."

After I finished the test, I handed it to the workers behind the desk and waited for my name to be called. I was soon brought to my room, and I waited anxiously.

Knock, knock! In came the doctor. "You are severely depressed."

I can't be. I am a pastor! We aren't supposed to have any problems.

She was right. I was severely depressed. I felt trapped in a sunless, colorless garden with dead flowers. I remember when my two-year-old, Dalton, would come into my room at 2:00 in the afternoon and say, "Da, seepy. Da, get up." I couldn't. I had no energy to face the day or get out of my bed. The only thing I felt I could do was sleep and cry on the inside. I was hurting so badly in the silent chamber of my soul that sometimes it was hard to breathe. That's how I felt, and there seemed to be no light at the end of the tunnel. I was living out the verse, "A crushed spirit dries up the bones" (Proverbs 17:22).

As a result of my depression, I isolated myself. Isolation and pastoring don't mix well together, so I decided that ministry wasn't for me. My inner critic whispered, *You are not good enough to be a pastor. Shame on you for being depressed.* I listened to the voice and applied to a high-class business in Rochester where I had always wanted to work. They hired me on the spot. I remember thinking, *Yes! I finally get to have a normal life.* I wanted to quit.

God had other plans.

He convinced me of those plans as I drove with my dad to pick up my mom from work. It was a ride I will never forget. After picking her up, I moved to the back seat. As Mom and Dad chatted with each other about their day, God's Spirit started talking to me. *Do not do it. Do not quit. If you quit, you will regret this for the rest of your life,* I sensed Him say.

This brief encounter with the Holy Spirit changed my outlook. It was as if the Spirit of God had flipped a switch in my spirit, and I went from being bent on quitting to being bent on not quitting. All these years later, I am so thankful I didn't quit.

Recognizing my broken spirit and deep depression, my place of ministry gave me a three-month sabbatical. I got away and had a total system reset. I spent a lot of time on the lakes of Okoboji, Iowa, where my mom and dad had a house, reflecting upon the behaviors and mindsets that had led to my breakdown. I learned that I had some wrong beliefs about mental illness. In addition, I became aware of some dysfunctional habits I had that led to my breakdown.

When I returned to the church three months later, I knew that I never wanted to sink that low again. I began to voraciously collect tools that would help me experience better mental health and spiritual well-being. I have been collecting these tools for over twenty years. I believe that period of my life was akin to what Nancy Koehn described as the "gathering years."[1] Gathering years are times when you don't feel that anything special is happening; however, looking back, you realize that you were being taught crucial lessons you can only appreciate with time. God processed me through that painful season. I want to share the insights I learned during those gathering years.

Mental Health: A Whole-Person Perspective

Before starting His ministry, Jesus exemplified a balanced life by developing in all aspects of His being. "And Jesus grew in wisdom and stature, and in favor with God and man" (Luke 2:52). Notice the four areas in which He grew:

- Mentally (wisdom)
- Physically (stature)
- Spiritually (favor with God)
- Relationally (favor with man)

In my experience, if you want to manage your mental health wisely, you need to develop a plan that includes all four dimensions—your whole being.

The Four Keys to Mental Health

This holistic approach to mental health is also seen in the words of Jesus: "'The most important one,' answered Jesus, 'is this: "Hear, O Israel: The Lord our God, the Lord is one. Love the Lord your God with all your heart and with all your soul and with all your mind and with all your strength'" (Mark 12:29–30).

Spiritual. The first key is the sacred one. This key focuses on your relationship and connection with Jesus because faith is the foundation of any mentally healthy person. "Love the Lord your God with all your heart and with all your soul." Chapters 1 through 8 will cover the spiritual key.

Mental. The second key is the psychological one that will show you tools that will increase your mental well-being. "Love the Lord your God . . . with all your mind." Chapters 9 through 15 will concentrate on this key.

Physical. The third key is the somatic one. "Love the Lord your God . . . with all your strength." This will focus on the physical part of your being. Chapters 16 through 21 will deal with this key.

Relational. The final key is the social key because to be mentally healthy, you need to be connected to others. "The second is this: 'Love your neighbor as yourself'" (Mark 12:31). Chapters 22 through 28 will focus on how to build healthy relationships.

The conclusion will wrap up what we have learned on our journey and give you a practical system for applying what you have learned.

Author Disclaimer

I am not a psychologist or trained mental health professional, and I don't pretend to be one. I am a pastor who is a fellow struggler. As a result, I want to encourage you to see a mental health professional if you are struggling. Often, the first step is to make an appointment with your primary care physician and tell them how you are feeling.

I also want to acknowledge that there are different degrees of mental health struggles. Some of you have had a much more difficult path than I have. My heart goes out to you. I may not totally understand what it is like to be in your shoes, but I do understand what it feels like to wrestle with making it through the day.

I also want you to understand that mental wellness is not a destination to be achieved but an ongoing path to walk. It is a lifelong journey, not a one-time event. At the end of this book, you will not be magically better. But you will have the tools to set off in the right direction. Progress, not perfection, is the goal. Ask the Lord to help you make using these tools a daily practice.

A Mental Health Journey

This book contains principles that will lead you to a higher level of mental well-being in Jesus. Please read each chapter slowly and process that chapter by doing the "Beyond the Book" exercises. Please do not skip this part. I pray that you don't just read this book but also apply its lessons to your life.

I am praying that by the end of this journey, you will look at your mental health in a whole new way. You will see it as one part of your overall health. You will see that to be as mentally healthy as possible, you must use all four keys. This whole-person perspective will help you experience the abundant life and divine joy Jesus promised. Imagine asking yourself every day, "How can I be a healthier, more whole person?"[2]

I am praying that working through this book will alter your life forever.

Let's begin our journey toward better mental health and spiritual well-being together!

BEYOND THE BOOK

Takeaway: The four keys are the foundations to moving toward higher summits of mental well-being.

Verse to memorize: "And Jesus grew in wisdom and stature, and in favor with God and man" (Luke 2:52).

Questions to consider: Have you treated mental health as a holistic issue in the past? Why or why not?

Reflections: _____

_____

_____

_____

Prayer: *Lord, Jesus, please give me a whole-person perspective on my mental health. Help me to see these four keys—spiritual, mental, physical, and relational—as interconnected and affecting each other. Please give me the discipline to commit to this journey and rise to a new level of health in my life. Amen.*

Application: Reflect on your current level of health in the four areas. Grade yourself on where you currently are (1 = Poor, 5 = Average, 10 = Outstanding):

Spiritual

1 ······ 2 ······ 3 ······ 4 ······ 5 ······ 6 ······ 7 ······ 8 ······ 9 ······ 10

Mental

1 ······ 2 ······ 3 ······ 4 ······ 5 ······ 6 ······ 7 ······ 8 ······ 9 ······ 10

Physical

1 ..... 2 ..... 3 ..... 4 ..... 5 ..... 6 ..... 7 ..... 8 ..... 9 10

Relational

1 ..... 2 ..... 3 ..... 4 ..... 5 ..... 6 ..... 7 ..... 8 ..... 9 10

PART ONE

The
Spiritual
Key

Jesus replied: "Love the Lord your God with all your heart."
Matthew 22:37

CHAPTER ONE

The Danger of Denial

My soul is downcast within me.

Lamentations 3:20

If I acknowledge my depression, I am admitting weakness! After being diagnosed with depression, I tried to deny it, like an ostrich that sticks its head in the sand. Ignoring it did not make it better; it made it worse.

Much worse!

God used my wife, Tammy, to stop the downward spiral of denial. We were staying at my parents' lake house in Okoboji, Iowa. It was beautiful weather—sunshine bounced off the blue lake, yellow finches darted in the sky, and the laughter of people on their boats could be heard for miles. Inwardly, however, I felt alone and trapped in a barren cave. I was wrestling with a decision. My pastoral overseers had recommended I take a sabbatical and some time off for healing.

"I am not sure what I should do. There is so much going on at church," I told Tammy.

The church was experiencing a season of upheaval, filled with division and strife. Those issues had led to many people leaving.

If I take the sabbatical, I will abandon them when they need me the most, I thought.

Tammy recognized my broken state better than I did. She was concerned about me because I wasn't myself. I had lost interest in things I normally enjoyed, such as reading, learning, and nature. She concluded I was not in the right mental place to lead the church.

"You can't take care of your own life right now," she said with firm conviction. "How do you expect to lead a church?"

"I am fine," I said abruptly.

"No, you are not." I sensed the Holy Spirit confirming her words as she said those uncomfortable truths: "You are not fine. You need help. Take the sabbatical. Quit living in denial."

That was the moment I acknowledged the truth about my mental health. I stepped out from under the dark cloud of denial into the bright light of the truth. By bringing it into the light and acknowledging it, I was able to begin the road to recovery.

Are you in a state of denial? In *The Attentive Life*, Leighton Ford writes, "Thoughts of darkness are not usually the most welcome. We prefer the bright and cheery. Kathleen Norris quotes a writer who said, 'The true religions of America are optimism and denial.' Yet moving out of denial into reality is absolutely essential."[1]

Has the time come for you to deny your denial and admit the truth of how you are doing?

As I moved out of denial, I started to research the nature of depression. I learned a lot of helpful things.

The Definition of Depression

Depression is:

> Depression is a mood disorder that causes a persistent feeling of sadness and loss of interest. Also called major depressive disorder or clinical depression, it affects how you feel, think, and behave and can lead to a variety of emotional and physical problems. You may have trouble doing normal day-to-day activities, and sometimes you may feel as if life isn't worth living.[2]

> In medical terms, depression is a serious illness that causes memory and thinking (cognitive), mood, physical, and behavior changes. It affects how you think, feel, eat, sleep, and act.[3]

Notice the phrase "medical terms." Depression is a medical issue, not a moral one. It often stems from forces you cannot control—biology, genetics, and traumatic events. It's a part of living in a fallen, broken world. Because of the fall, people experience brokenness in diverse ways: body, spirit, relationships, and the mind.

At first, I didn't understand this. I thought that since I wrestled with depression, I was a bad Christian. I felt as though I had done something wrong to deserve it. Once I learned that depression was a medical issue, like heart disease, diabetes, or hypothyroidism, I felt free to acknowledge it and no longer saw it as stemming from my "badness."

The Depression of David

In my journey of accepting my diagnosis, one of the most encouraging truths I discovered is that several giants of the faith wrestled with depression. We will talk about many of them in this book. One of those who struggled was David. David's story combines mountains and valleys. One of the valleys he experienced was depression. Psalm 102 highlights his struggle. From this passage, Michael Lyles, in the *Soul Care Bible,* shares six signs of depression that David exhibited:[4]

Crying. "For I eat ashes as my food and mingle my drink with tears" (Psalm 102:9). David was so depressed that he wept, and those droplets of tears fell into his drink. Breathless weeping often accompanies gloomy despair. These tears of sadness often come as a series of cresting waves on the seashore.

Physical. "My bones burn like glowing embers" (Psalm 102:3). David's depression didn't just affect his mood—it also affected his body. It caused him to have physical symptoms. It can affect us in the same way. It can lead to a weakened immune system, chronic pain, and sleep disturbances, to name a few.

Purpose. "For my days vanish like smoke. . . . My heart is blighted and withered like grass" (Psalm 102:3–4). David lost sight of his purpose during his depression. In the dark clouds of depression, we, too, can lose our sense of direction and begin to drift aimlessly instead of living purposefully. Has that happened to you? Have you become like an aimless piece of driftwood floating wherever the tide takes you?

Nutrition. "I forget to eat my food" (Psalm 102:4). David neglected to eat because he was so depressed. Depression can affect people's food habits. It leads some people to overeat. They eat past their capacity for the dopamine hit it provides. Others will pick at their food or skip meals entirely.

Loneliness. "I am like a desert owl, like an owl among the ruins" (Psalm 102:6). Imagine a feathery, wide-eyed owl alone in the desert. That's how David felt in his season of depression. Depression can be a lonely struggle. One of the reasons it can lead to loneliness is because socializing takes energy. When people are depressed, they don't have much energy. So they choose to stay home instead of going to their small group. The very thing they are doing—isolating themselves—is the thing that is making them more depressed. It is a vicious cycle. Has depression made you a lonely owl?

Sleep. "I lie awake" (Psalm 102:7). David's depression kept him up at night. Is depression having an impact on the quality of your sleep? Do you wake up early in the morning and are unable to get back to sleep? Do you find yourself wrestling with fatigue all day long?

The *First* Step to Managing Depression

Is it possible that God led you to this book to help you see the mental anguish you are in and find the courage to admit it?

To begin healing yourself, you have to admit that you're in pain. The denial reflex is especially strong in successful people, and to break through that barrier takes courage, but mostly it requires an effort at awareness that keeps denial from occurring automatically. Ask yourself questions like "What's the worst that can happen to me if I admit that everything *isn't* okay?"[5]

Is it time for you to admit that everything is not okay? Is it time for you to acknowledge the reality of your mental well-being—or lack of it?

Jesus said, "Blessed are the poor in spirit, for theirs is the kingdom of heaven" (Matthew 5:3). Why did Jesus call the poor in spirit blessed? Because they recognized their neediness before God and asked for His help. God helps those who ask for His help. Is it time for you to get help?

Under His Training

During the summer of 2002, I discovered a quote from Andrew Murray that helped me accept my pain and see it as an anvil for God to use to shape my soul. After reading it, I also began to wonder if God might be able to use this experience for me to help others someday. Little did I know that I would write a book about that concept. In times of trouble say:

> *First*, He brought me here, it is by His will I am in this strait place: in that fact I will rest. *Next*, He will keep me here in His love, and give me grace to behave as His child. *Then*, He will make the trial a blessing, teaching me the lessons He intends me to learn, and working in me the grace He means to bestow. *Last*, In His good time He can bring me out again—how and when He knows. Let me say I am here, (1) By God's appointment, (2) In His keeping, (3) Under His training, (4) For His time.[6]

BEYOND THE BOOK

Takeaway: Denial keeps you locked in the dungeon of despair.

Verse to memorize: "Then you will know the truth, and the truth will set you free" (John 8:32).

Questions to consider: Am I denying the truth about my current mental health? If so, why?

Reflections: _____

_____

_____

_____

_____

Prayer: *Lord, I acknowledge that my tendency to deny the truth about my mental well-being runs deep. Please help me get out of this destructive rut so that I can start down the path to healing. Please give me the courage to be honest with You, others, and most of all myself. Help me to move out of the land of denial and into the land of freedom that the truth brings. Amen.*

Application: Are you wrestling with the symptoms of depression David had?

Y or N: Crying and sadness

Y or N: Physical ailments

Y or N: Loss of purpose

Y or N: Dietary changes

Y or N: Loneliness

Y or N: Sleep disturbances

CHAPTER TWO

The Victory of Vulnerability

We were under great pressure, far beyond our ability to endure, so that we despaired of life itself.

2 Corinthians 1:8

After being diagnosed with severe anxiety and depression, I began to dwell on a self-imposed island of isolation. *I am the only pastor wrestling with depression,* I erroneously thought. Since I didn't know of any other pastors wrestling with depression, I incorrectly assumed I was the only one.

This misbelief was shattered one day as I walked through the rows of books at the Rochester Public Library. I was in search of answers, of hope. I felt defeated and lost. I felt all alone. Amid the tranquil library, where people sat quietly studying at their tables, God gave me a life jacket of hope.

As I was journeying through the rows of books, a tape series on anxiety and depression literally fell off the shelf and into my cart. (Do you remember cassette tapes?) *What's this?* I thought. I read the course description on the back. *This looks interesting.*

Upon returning home, I listened to it. On one side of the tape was a teaching on how to cope with anxiety and depression. On the other side was a testimony of a pastor who had wrestled with anxiety and depression.

I am not the only one, I began to believe as I listened to his testimony. *Other pastors have wrestled with depression.*

Learning that I was not alone was a major step forward in my mental well-being. As that truth entered my mind, hope began to rise in my heart. I thank God for that pastor who was vulnerable enough to share his struggle. It was a ray of hope for me.

I pray this book will do for you what that pastor's testimony did for me. I hope that hearing my story will help you feel less alone. In addition, I pray that God will give you the courage to be vulnerable and share your story with others. Your story may be their ray of hope.

The Perception of Isolation

The prophet Elijah went through severe depression after a momentous victory on Mount Carmel. One of the interesting comments he makes during that season of depression is, "I have been very zealous for the LORD God Almighty. The Israelites have rejected your covenant, torn down your altars, and put your prophets to death with the sword. *I am the only one left*, and now they are trying to kill me too" (1 Kings 19:10, emphasis added).

Notice his perception of isolation. He felt alone in his battle; however, here is the real question: Was it true? Was he the only one left?

No!

"Yet I reserve seven thousand in Israel—all whose knees have not bowed down to Baal and whose mouths have not kissed him" (1 Kings 19:18).

Elijah felt alone, but there were seven thousand others. The moral of the story is that our feelings are not facts. They are surges of neurochemicals that must be filtered through the truth of God's Word.

Isolation and Illness Cycle

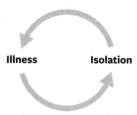

When I am walking through a season of depression, I tend to isolate myself. I don't feel like socializing . . . so I don't. The thing I need the most is a Christian community—yet I avoid it. This turns into a self-defeating cycle: The more mentally ill I feel, the more I isolate myself. The more I isolate myself, the more ill I feel. Round and round the cycle goes.

Are you familiar with this illness/isolation cycle?

Now, please do not misunderstand me. I am not saying that we don't need solitude. There is a difference between isolation and solitude. John Mark Comer wrote, "Solitude is engagement; isolation is escape. Solitude is safety; isolation is danger. Solitude is how you open yourself up to God; isolation is painting a target on your back for the tempter."[1]

We all need solitude. The danger comes when solitude drifts into isolation.

The Loneliness of Depression

One of the reasons that depression can be lonely for Christians is that their church family shames them instead of helping them. Amy Simpson, author of *Troubled Minds*, writes:

> The suffering of mental illness, whether for the afflicted or for their families, is typically marked by isolation. When people desperately need to experience the love and empathy of their fellow human beings and to know that their Creator has not abandoned them, many reach out and are shocked to touch the church's painfully cold shoulder. Others fear the church's rejection enough to hide their struggles and not risk exposure at all.[2]

According to Simpson, one of the main reasons for this loneliness in churches is what she calls the "victorious Christian living" paradigm, which believes: "If you are a good Christian, you will live in victory. You won't have problems. If you have enough faith, read the Bible enough, and pray enough, you won't have problems like mental illness."[3]

The logical conclusion to this faulty worldview is clear—if you have problems—like mental illness—it is your fault. You have done something wrong to deserve it. Perhaps you are not spiritual enough. Perhaps you don't have enough faith. Because of this faulty mindset, people who are struggling keep silent instead of reaching out for help.

At the church where I pastor, we have intentionally avoided this victorious Christian living paradigm. Please do not misunderstand me. I am not saying we shouldn't have faith and believe God for great things. But what I am saying is that we live in a broken world and that brokenness shows up in our lives in different ways. At those times, we should be able to share our struggles with our church family and receive their help and hope instead of judgment and shame. "The ground is level at the foot of the cross."[4]

"Therefore confess your sins to each other and pray for each other so that you may be healed" (James 5:16). Note that healing comes from admitting our struggles to others, not hiding them. We need, of course, to be selective in who we share our struggles with. Confession, not suppression, is the answer.

The Bridge of Vulnerability

Earlier, I shared the feeling of being stranded on an island of isolation due to my depression. Thankfully, I discovered the bridge of vulnerability that led me off that island. When I began to share my story with others, warts and all, I saw that others seemed to receive permission to take off their masks and share their stories. I learned that victory comes from vulnerability. Modeling vulnerability, the apostle Paul wrote, "We were under great pressure, far beyond our ability to endure, so that *we despaired of life itself*" (2 Corinthians 1:8, emphasis added).

In *What's So Amazing About Grace?*, Philip Yancey shares the lessons he learned from observing an Alcoholics Anonymous group that met on Tuesday nights in the basement of the church he attended.

First, he noticed the lack of a pecking order. Millionaires would freely interact with unemployed dropouts, and vice versa. The group's culture was devoid of spiritual elitism and self-righteousness.

That really moved him.

His big takeaway, however, was, "They began with radical honesty and ended with radical dependence."[5] Unlike many Christians who come to church and put on airs, they came with unmistakable dependence on God. They knew that to get better, they needed outside help—from God and other members of the group. "But this happened that we might not rely on ourselves but on God, who raises the dead" (2 Corinthians 1:9).

May God help us to learn the lessons of the Tuesday night group! May we ask God to remove our self-righteousness and spiritual arrogance. May we instead be known for our radical honesty, because as psychologist Joan Borysenko said, "Vulnerability—being imperfect—is what makes us human, authentic, and lovable."[6]

May we also be known for radical dependency. "Trust in the LORD with all your heart and lean not on your own understanding; in all your ways submit to him, and he will make your paths straight" (Proverbs 3:5–6).

Is the Holy Spirit nudging you to cross the bridge of vulnerability?

BEYOND THE BOOK

Takeaway: Victory comes from vulnerability. The bridge of vulnerability leads you off the island of isolation. When you cross that bridge, you inspire others to do the same.

Verse to memorize: "We were under great pressure, far beyond our ability to endure, so that we despaired of life itself. Indeed, we felt we had received the sentence of death. But this happened that we might not rely on ourselves but on God, who raises the dead" (2 Corinthians 1:8–9).

Questions to consider: Can you relate to the illness/isolation cycle? How has it affected you?

Reflections:

Prayer: *Lord, sometimes I feel all alone in my mental illness, tempted to suffer in silence. Please give me the courage to cross the bridge of vulnerability, knowing that my vulnerability could be the catalyst for others to admit their struggle and seek help. Please show me fellow strugglers with whom I can link arms and do life together. Amen.*

Application: Find a safe person with whom you can share your struggle. Or find a mental health support group. Don't listen to the lie of depression that tries to tell you that you are the only one. Remember that victory comes from vulnerability.

CHAPTER THREE

The Stigma of Shame

Darkness is my closest friend.
Psalm 88:18

"What words come to your mind when you think of someone struggling with cancer?"

The leader of our church's mental health support ministry posed that question to the group as they sat in a circle sipping their hot coffee.

One member blurted out, "Champion." Synergy began to occur among the group. The leader walked over to the whiteboard and wrote "champion."

"Hero," another person added.

"Survivor." At this point, the group's energy was optimistic. The leader posed a new question.

"What comes to people's minds when they think of mental illness?" The entire tone of the group changed.

"Crazy."

"Cooky."

"Lunatic"

"Wacko."

"Weak."

Is there any wonder why those who are wrestling with a mental illness often don't tell anyone or seek help? They don't want to be labeled as weak or crazy. Why is it that people are said to be heroic if they wrestle with a physical illness but defective if they wrestle with a mental one? The lesson is clear: "We live in a culture that stigmatizes certain types of brokenness more than others."[1]

What makes one kind of brokenness good and another bad? Aren't we all broken in diverse ways?

The Stigma of Shame

The US surgeon general called the stigma of mental health "the most formidable obstacle to the future progress in the arena of mental illness and health."[2]

A major reason for this label is that the mental health stigma stops people from getting the help they need.

Is it stopping you?

One of the roots of the stigma is shame. People feel ashamed for experiencing mental brokenness. Are you stuck in the trap of shame today? Do you feel ashamed of your mental health struggles? If so, that is not coming from God—it is coming from Satan, who the Bible says, "For the accuser of our brothers and sisters, who accuses them before our God day and night, has been hurled down" (Revelation 12:10).

You may wonder, "What is the difference between guilt and shame?"

Guilt and Shame

Guilt says that you did something wrong; however, God will forgive you if you repent of your sin and ask Him to forgive you. "If we confess our sins, he is faithful and just and will forgive us our sins and purify us from all unrighteousness" (1 John 1:9).

Shame says, "You are wrong, and nothing can fix it." In *Tired of Trying to Measure Up*, Jeff VanVonderen wrote,

Shame is the belief or mindset that something is wrong with you. It's something you can live with and not necessarily be aware of. It's not that you feel bad about your behavior, it's that you sense or believe you are deficient, defective, and worthless as a human being.[3]

People who wrestle with mental illness can get stuck in the trap of shame in which they feel worthless and defective because of their illness.

The Source of Shame

According to Lewis Smedes, shame comes from three sources:[4]

1. Unaccepting parents. These parents put conditions on their love:

- "I will love you if you get good grades."
- "I will love you if you make good choices."
- "I will love you if you are a good Christian man or woman."

Are these the kind of messages you received from your family of origin? If you performed well, you were loved—if you didn't, love was withheld. Did you get the message that love was conditional and had strings attached? If so, you may have developed a shame-based worldview.

Before we move on, my goal in sharing this is not to blame your parents. They were probably doing the best they could with what they knew at the time. There are no perfect parents—me included. Rather than blaming parents, our goal is to self-reflect on the root of shame orientation.

2. Secular culture. Modern advertisements condition us to believe we are not enough:

- You are not thin enough.
- You don't earn enough.
- You're not powerful enough.
- You don't have enough stuff.

They seek to make us feel defective so that we will buy their products. Is this strategy working?

3. Graceless religion. Another word for graceless religion is legalism, which believes you gain God's approval by following all the rules. Legalism leads people to think that if they obey God's law, He will approve of them. If they don't, He won't. Legalism often leads people to jump on the treadmill of more. They feel as if they need to pray more, serve more, give more, and do more. As a result, they become spiritually tired.

The Antidote to Shame

If shame is the problem, then grace is the solution. "For it is by grace you have been saved, through faith—and this is not from yourselves, it is the gift of God" (Ephesians 2:8). We begin our walk with God by grace through faith. Salvation is not something we earn through good works; we receive it through faith in Jesus. Grace is the unmerited favor of God. If you've earned it, it is not grace. Philip Yancey defines grace this way:

> Grace means there's nothing we can do to make God love us more.
> . . . And grace means there is nothing we can do to make God love
> us less. . . . Grace means that God already loves us as much as an
> infinite God can possibly love.[5]

"Is grace a license to disobey God?" you ask.

No. "What shall we say, then? Shall we go on sinning so that grace may increase? By no means! We are those who have died to sin; how can we live in it any longer?" (Romans 6:1–2). Grace is not an excuse to sin; it's the power that leads to loving obedience.

The late Timothy Keller wrote that John 14:21–23 is the key to understanding the relationship of law and grace:

> Whoever has my commands and keeps them is the one who loves
> me. The one who loves me will be loved by my Father, and I too
> will love them and show myself to them. . . . Anyone who loves

me will obey my teaching. My Father will love them, and we will come to them and make our home with them.

Commenting on that verse, Keller writes:

> The gospel transforms obedience to God's commands from a legalistic means of acquiring salvation to a loving response to a received salvation. Obedience to God's law, flowing out of gospel grace, becomes a way to know, resemble, delight, and love the one who saved us at infinite cost to himself.[6]

We obey God's commands not to earn His love but because we are already in a loving relationship with Him. Obedience is a way of expressing our love for Him, and grace enables us to live a lifestyle of joyful, loving obedience.

Understanding God's unconditional love and grace was a very healing force during my depression. I came to understand that God didn't love me less when I was depressed. He didn't love me more when I was mentally well. Unlike human love, which can be fickle, God's love is fixed. It's not dependent on our inconsistent behavior but on His consistent nature.

His unconditional love was expressed for us on the cross. "But God demonstrates his own love for us in this: While we were still sinners, Christ died for us" (Romans 5:8). He didn't wait until we had arrived to express His love. No, He loved us while we were yet sinners. That's unconditional love. That's grace.

As I began to better understand God's unconditional love, as expressed on the cross, I wrote a grace affirmation that I repeated to myself many times throughout the day. "My value and worth come not from my performance but from Jesus' performance for me on the cross."

That's grace!

BEYOND THE BOOK

Takeaway: Shame knocked on the door. Grace answered, and there was no one there.

Verse to memorize: "Therefore, there is now no condemnation for those who are in Christ Jesus" (Romans 8:1).

Questions to consider: Am I listening to the voice of shame in my life? Or am I listening to the voice of grace?

Reflections:

_____

_____

_____

_____

_____

Prayer: *Lord, help me to recognize the suffocating whispers of shame when they falsely communicate that I am defective and unworthy. I choose to listen to Your voice of grace, not Satan's words of shame. Remind me that You love me based on Your loving nature and that I can do nothing to make You love me any more or less. Plant in me a more profound desire to obey Your commands, not to earn Your love but as a way of expressing my love back to You. Amen.*

Application: Where do your shame messages come from?

   Y or N: Unaccepting parents
   Y or N: Secular culture
   Y or N: Graceless religion

CHAPTER FOUR

The Cost of Control

Be still, and know that I am God.

Psalm 46:10

"Are you questioning our marriage?" I asked my wife on our anniversary in 2019. As we played miniature golf, I noticed the radiant afternoon we were experiencing. The sky was clear, and I could feel the sun's warmth on my cheeks; however, my wife seemed distant and cold. She had been that way for a while.

"Yes," she replied.

Panic filled my heart.

Struggling in our marriage was not new. You could not find two people who are more different from each other. Our different upbringings, personalities, and viewpoints caused us to clash often. We had gone to many counselors, but this was the first time she hinted at the "D" word—divorce.

After much talking and counseling, she moved out of our house and into an apartment. We were separated for over a year. The low point came when we met with a mediator to end our marriage. We sat across the long rectangular table from each other, more distant and lonelier than ever, and split up our stuff with the help of a mediator.

The Illusion of Control

During this marriage storm, I came to understand something called "the illusion of control," a phrase coined by psychologist Ellen Langer.[1] This is believing you have control over things that you don't. God used this storm, the outcome of which was out of my control, to break my illusion. Specifically, He taught me three imperatives for shattering the illusion of control.

Define what you can control. There are things in life we can control and things we can't. Chris Hodges labels these two categories as facts of life and problems. "Facts of life are matters you cannot always, if ever, control. Problems, on the other hand, can usually be fixed. It's important to learn to discern the difference and live accordingly to live in peace and harmony."[2]

Accept what you can't control. Anger. Frustration. Resentment. Those words are what I was feeling as I vented to a counselor about the struggles of Tammy and me. After vomiting my pain on him, he said something that caught me off guard: "Accept it."

I am not going to accept it. I am going to fight it, I thought.

He explained what accepting the situation meant. As he did, his words began to make more sense. He was not saying I should approve of or agree with the problem, but rather accept it as being out of my control and place it in God's to-do box. Once I did this, I could switch my focus from complaining about what I couldn't control to working on the things within my control—mainly my faith, attitude, and choices.

"God, grant me the serenity to accept the things I cannot change, courage to change the things I can, and wisdom to know the difference," says the Serenity Prayer.[3]

Amen to that!

Surrender to God's ultimate control. As human beings, our circle of control is very minute. God's circle of control is infinitely vast. He is the sovereign King over everything. "The LORD has established his throne in heaven, and his kingdom rules overall" (Psalm 103:19).

Prayer is the link between our finiteness and His infiniteness. As we connect to God in prayer, we give Him our troubles. "Cast all your anxiety on him because he cares for you" (1 Peter 5:7)—and He gives us His love, joy, and peace.

What a delightful exchange!

If we have this incredible privilege to talk to the King every day, why do so few people do it? One reason is because of self-reliance. That's my story. In my early twenties, I became a fan of the self-help movement. I read countless books on it and listened to many of its teachings. Though it had some benefits, one of its major setbacks was that it planted an erroneous seed in my mind: If it is to be, it's up to me. I developed a self-reliant stance toward life and ministry. That made me often feel like Atlas with the world's weight on my shoulders. Stress, pressure, and anxiety were my daily companions. I believe this self-reliant attitude was one of the contributing factors to my breakdown in 2002.

This self-reliant mode came to my awareness one day as I read the book *Experiencing God*. I had gone to a local park to hide from people because I felt as if my problems were caving in on me. I felt hopeless. Powerless. Helpless. A ray of hope came as I read the following words:

> Some would define a servant like this: "A servant is one who finds out what his master wants him to do, and then he does it." The human concept of a servant is that a servant goes to the master and says, "Master, what do you want me to do?" The master tells him, and the servant goes off *by himself* and does it. That is not the biblical concept of a servant of God. Being a servant of God is different than being a servant of a human master. A servant of a human master works *for* his master. God, however, works *through* his servants.[4]

To sum it up, the worldly view of a servant is someone who does the work in their own strength. The biblical view of a servant is someone who allows God to do the work through them with His unlimited strength.

As I sat in that park listening to the birds chirping and hearing the gurgling sounds of water in the passing stream, I had a moment of clarity. *I am following the worldly way of service. No wonder I am depleted. My strength is limited; God's strength, however, is unlimited.*

I vowed to make a change. I vowed to quit working for God and, instead, allow Him to work through me. As a result, I began to see my primary role as walking with Jesus, knowing that out of the overflow of that relationship, Jesus would do His work through me. I pivoted from the attitude of "If it is to be, it's up to me" to "If it is to be, it's up to Christ working through me."

As I did, my prayer life became stronger, richer, and deeper. I quit hoping for time to pray, and I began making time for it.

One of the most helpful prayer practices I developed was praying the Jesus Prayer: Not my will, but thy will be done. Through this prayer, I exchanged my wishes for God's will. This further helped me surrender the illusion of control and sync with the sovereign control of God.

> To grow spiritually is to allow one's whole life to come more and more under the lordship of Christ. Spiritual growth is the process by which this happens. To put it another way, spiritual growth means that our lives are increasingly directed by the Holy Spirit.[5]

Another benefit of expanding your prayer life is that it leads to a healthier brain. In their book *How God Changes the Brain*, the authors write:

> Activities involving meditation and intensive prayer permanently strengthen neural functioning in specific parts of the brain that are involved with lowering anxiety and depression, enhancing social awareness and empathy, and improving cognitive and intellectual functioning.[6]

If you want a healthier brain, pray!

Moreover, the longer you pray, the better your brain health will be.

> Neurologically, we have found that the longer one prays or meditates, the more changes occur in the brain. Five minutes of prayer once

a week may have little effect, but forty minutes of daily practice, over a period of years, will bring permanent changes to the brain.[7]

The Prayer Meeting

I wanted to save my marriage, so I asked Tammy to attend a marriage retreat. She quickly responded, "No. I am done."

I called a prayer meeting at church. About twenty people came and asked God to save my marriage. It lasted about two hours.

Tammy sent me a surprising text the next day: "I am willing to go to the marriage retreat with you."

God had performed a miracle.

I am convinced that the prayer meeting saved my marriage.

A few weeks later, we attended that marriage conference, and the momentum of our marriage changed. We went from drifting away from one another to moving toward each other. About a year later, we renewed our vows in Cozumel, Mexico.

BEYOND THE BOOK

Takeaway: Through prayer, we let go of the illusion of control and join hands with the One in ultimate control.

Verse to memorize: "Do not be anxious about anything, but in every situation, by prayer and petition, with thanksgiving, present your requests to God" (Philippians 4:6).

Question to consider: In what areas of your life are you buying into the illusion of control?

Reflections:

_____

_____

_____

Prayer: *Lord, thank You for being sovereign and in control. Even when my life seems out of control, I trust that You are in control. By faith, I let go of the illusion of control. I chose to stop trying to exert power where I have none and instead focus on what is within my control—myself. I decide to exchange pressure for peace by lifting my burdens into Your loving arms through prayer. Amen.*

Application: Ponder a situation you are fretting about. Identify the things you can control and ask for God's guidance to resolve them. Discover the things you can't control and ask God to help you accept them. Leave them in His to-do box.

Things I CAN Control	Things I CAN'T Control

CHAPTER FIVE

The Impact of Identity

Therefore, if anyone is in Christ, the new creation has come: The old has gone, the new is here!

2 Corinthians 5:17

A couple years into our church plant, two families got into a heated conflict. Overnight, they went from being great friends to being at sharp odds with one another. The conflict stemmed from some hurtful words spoken between them. Afterward, battle lines were drawn. One of the sides went on a campaign to get others to join their side and oppose the others. The circle of conflict spread to the whole church. When we got together for a group meeting, everyone could feel the tension in the air. People hung out in little cliques and whispered about the other side.

Due to my youth and inexperience, I did not respond wisely to the conflict. My attempts to resolve it only made it worse. People began to leave the church in droves. As a result, I thought that our church wouldn't be around in six months.

Because our young church seemed to be falling apart, I fell apart. I had erroneously received my identity from the ministry. If it was going well, I felt great. If it wasn't, I felt defeated.

Looking back, my core problem was that I got my identity from what I did rather than who I was in Jesus. I turned ministry into idolatry, letting its apparent success or failure define me. This is dangerous.

> Once the enemy, the devil, has a person deeply convinced of the lie that something or someone other than Jesus Christ is the foundation of life, he is open prey for the crippling pain of misbelief. Our lives hold meaning because God loves us and because we are His.[1]

I vowed to no longer get my identity from anything other than Jesus. As I went on that journey to firmly anchor my identity in Christ, I asked a few questions.

What Is Identity?

In their book *Defined,* the Kendrick brothers define identity this way: "The word *identity* describes who you are in totality. It's the real truth about the real you."[2]

They go on to say that there are two big questions in life: *Who is God?* and *Who am I?*[3]

Identity answers the question, "Who am I?"

What are some identity traps? What is the foundation of your identity? Who or what are you allowing to define you? Is it one of the following identity traps?

I am how I look. Do you get your sense of worth and value from your physical appearance? When you look good, you feel good, though that doesn't happen nearly as often as you would like.

I am who my bank account says I am. Do you get your value from your net worth? Is your scorecard your bank account? Do you consider big purchases to be your life milestones?

I am what I have achieved. Do you get your identity from the trophies you have? Do your accomplishments define you? Are you defined by the titles or degrees attached to your name?

I am who others say I am. Do you get your identity from what others think about you? Sociologist George Herbert Meade coined the phrase "generalized other."[4] This is the group of people you have in your mind whose evaluation of you determines whether you are a failure or success.

I am what I have done in the past. Is your identity linked to your past? Are you struggling to get past it? Do you define yourself by your mistakes?

I am my illness. Does your illness define you? "I am so ADHD." Do you find yourself saying, "I do _____ because I am so anxious"?

Have you fallen into one of these identity traps?

What Is the Biblical Alternative?

Then Jesus came from Galilee to the Jordan to be baptized by John. But John tried to deter him, saying, "I need to be baptized by you, and do you come to me?" Jesus replied, "Let it be so now; it is proper for us to do this to fulfill all righteousness." Then John consented. As soon as Jesus was baptized, he went up out of the water. At that moment heaven was opened, and he saw the Spirit of God descending like a dove and alighting on him. And a voice from heaven said, "This is my Son, whom I love; with him I am well pleased."

Matthew 3:13–17

Carefully notice that at the beginning of Jesus' ministry, the Father affirmed that Jesus was His beloved Son. He also affirmed that He loved Jesus and was well pleased with Him. Even more telling is *when* He did this. When the Father affirmed Jesus, He was an unknown. He had not done all the things He would later be remembered for:

- He hadn't gone to the cross.
- He hadn't walked on water.
- He hadn't fed five thousand.
- He hadn't raised the dead.

- He hadn't healed a bunch of sick people.
- He hadn't cleared the temple.

He was an unknown. Yet that didn't matter. In his book *Transforming Leadership*, Leighton Ford writes that Jesus, "affirmed God as the only source of his identity."[5] Imagine if we followed His example! When people ask about us, imagine if we didn't respond by saying, "I am a librarian. I am a janitor. I am a doctor." But rather, "I am the one Jesus loves."[6]

Does Satan attack our identity? One of the most fundamental truths of the Bible, if you are a Jesus follower, is that you have an enemy. He is known as Satan or the adversary. He comes to "steal and kill and destroy" (John 10:10). One of the primary ways he does that is to blind us to who we are in Jesus. This is not a new tactic. He tried the same thing on Jesus.

> Then Jesus was led by the Spirit into the wilderness to be tempted by the devil. After fasting forty days and forty nights, he was hungry. The tempter came to him and said, *"If you are the Son of God, tell these stones to become bread."*
>
> Matthew 4:1–3, emphasis added

Note that key phrase: "If you are the Son of God." In the verses right before these, we see the Father affirming Jesus as His beloved Son (see Matthew 3:16–17). Satan counters the Father's words. He tries to get Jesus to forget who He is. He uses the same trick on God's children today. Has the enemy stolen your identity?

Who does God say I am? One of the biggest decisions in life is this: Who or what are you going to allow to define you? Where will you look for your identity? If you look to something or someone other than Jesus, you are opening yourself up to massive pain and crippling disappointment. Here is the truth: You are not what others say you are. You are not your past. You are not your bank account.

You are who God says you are.

Take a moment and declare with faith, "I am who I AM says that I am" (see Exodus 3:14). And He says that:

- I am God's beloved child. "The Spirit you received does not make you slaves, so that you live in fear again; rather, the Spirit you received brought about your adoption to sonship. And by him we cry, 'Abba, Father'" (Romans 8:15).
- I am fearfully and wonderfully made. "I praise you because I am fearfully and wonderfully made; your works are wonderful, I know that full well" (Psalm 139:14).
- I am uniquely gifted by God. "For this reason I remind you to fan into flame the gift of God, which is in you through the laying on of my hands" (2 Timothy 1:6).
- I am loved. "This is love: not that we loved God, but that he loved us and sent his Son as an atoning sacrifice for our sins" (1 John 4:10).
- I am a work of art. "For we are God's handiwork, created in Christ Jesus to do good works, which God prepared in advance for us to do" (Ephesians 2:10).

May you not allow your illness to define you. But rather, may you look to Jesus and Jesus alone to answer the question, Who am I? May you remember that you are infinitely special because of who you are in Christ and, "To be loved by God is the highest relationship, the highest achievement, and the highest position in life."[7]

BEYOND THE BOOK

Takeaway: I am who I AM says that I am (see Exodus 3:14).

Verse to memorize: "Now if we are children, then we are heirs—heirs of God and co-heirs with Christ, if indeed we share in his sufferings so that we may also share in his glory" (Romans 8:17).

Question to consider: What would be different in your life if you truly believed that your core identity is being a child of God?

Reflections:

Prayer: *Lord, the enemy has attempted to steal my identity. At times his tactics have worked, and I have gotten my identity from the wrong place. By faith, today I affirm that my core identity is not what I do or what others say, but who I am in You. I am Your beloved child. I chose to get my identity from the firm foundation of Your Word, not the fickle opinion of people. Today, I declare from the roof tops, "I am who I AM says that I am."*

Application: I get my identity from:

   T or F: How I look.

   T or F: Who my bank account says I am.

   T or F: What I achieve.

   T or F: Who others say I am.

   T or F: What I have done in the past.

   T or F: My illness.

   T or F: Who I AM says that I am.

CHAPTER SIX

The Healing of Hope

My hope is in you.

Psalm 39:7

If I run my car into that tree, my pain will be over!

Suicidal thoughts raced through my mind as I drove home from basketball practice in the eleventh grade. Looking back, I now realize I was going through my first depressive episode. I felt devoid of hope. Emotionally, I felt as though a dark cloud of despair was hovering over my life. The stress and pressures of life were caving in on me like a C-clamp.

Back in the early 1990s, when this situation happened, mental illness was like the elephant in the room that no one talked about. Because of this atmosphere of silence, I did not get treatment. This is dangerous because untreated depression is one of the leading causes of suicide.[1]

By God's grace, I didn't act upon that thought. I made it through that first bout of depression with the loving support of my family and the gracious compassion of Jesus.

I pray you will never act upon a suicidal thought or urge, but rather talk to someone who can help you, such as a doctor, a teacher, or a pastor. Don't suffer in silence.

It's okay not to be okay, just don't be not okay alone! Tell someone.

The Hope Bucket

Imagine that your soul is like a bucket filled with water, and the water in the bucket represents hope. How full is your bucket of hope today?

- Full? Are you brimming to the top with hope? Almost overflowing?
- Halfway? Do you have just enough hope to make it through the day but none to spare?
- Empty? Has your bucket been knocked over and emptied?

Back in the summer of 2002, not only was my hope bucket empty, but I felt as dry as a prickly cactus. Thankfully, during that time the Lord pointed out a phrase in Psalm 23 that filled me with hope. "Even though I walk *through* the darkest valley" (Psalm 23:4, emphasis added). Did you see it? We walk *through* the dark valley.

It is a temporary state, not a permanent residence.

I came to believe that I wouldn't always feel sad, depressed, or discouraged. One day I would feel better. This revelation was like the first drop of water in my hope bucket. I soon learned five other things that filled me with hope.

The therapy of trust. The essence of being a Christian is trusting in Jesus. Every day that I wrestled with depression, I had a decision to make—trust God or not trust Him. My faith grew during this dark season. I learned that faith is not just believing God for great things but also trusting Him in the storms. That reminds me of a story I once read.

A young man from China had a beloved horse that ran away.

His neighbors said, "I am so sorry for your bad fortune."

His dad responded differently. "What makes you so sure this isn't a blessing?"

A *blessing*? One day his horse returned.

"Congratulations," his neighbors exclaimed.

"What makes you sure this isn't a disaster?" his dad asked. Celebrating his good fortune, the young man took his stallion for a ride. On that ride, the young man fell off the horse and fractured his hip.

"That is terrible," the neighbors mumbled.

"What makes you sure this isn't a blessing?" his father inquired.

Sometime later, war broke out, and all the young men were required to go and fight. Because of his broken hip, this young man did not go. Nine out of ten of those young men who went died in battle. This young man survived because of his broken hip.[2]

Can you relate to this young man? Because of your mental health challenges, are you mourning the loss of energy? Vitality? Zest for living? If so, please ask God to help you trust Him even when you don't understand your current reality, believing that "the LORD works out everything to its proper end" (Proverbs 16:4).

The remedy of remembering. One of the ways to build your trust in God is to recall His past faithfulness. David models this. Recall when he was facing Goliath. From a human perspective, that situation seemed hopeless; however, David was filled with hope. Why? He recalled God's past faithfulness. As he faced Goliath, he remembered the "giants" in the past that God had slain. He said, "The LORD who rescued me from the paw of the lion and the paw of the bear will rescue me from the hand of this Philistine" (1 Samuel 17:37).

What if you were to follow his example? What if you were to take out a notepad and write down the difficult situations you have faced that God got you through? Might recalling God's past faithfulness fill your hope bucket? The same God who helped you overcome the giants of the past will empower you to overcome your current and future ones.

The art of anticipation. Since God has been faithful in the past, you can anticipate His faithfulness now. "Perhaps this breakdown will lead to a breakthrough," you declare in faith. Charles Spurgeon, a British pastor, came to anticipate God's blessings when he went through a season of depression. He tells about it in one of his lectures, "The Minister's Fainting Fits." In it, he described how he often experienced depression before a breakthrough. "Before any great achievement, some measure of depression is very usual. . . . This depression came over me whenever the Lord is preparing a larger blessing for my ministry."[3] Is it possible that God has a blessing for you on the other side of your depression?

The power of persistence. Persistence is moving forward when you feel like giving up. "Let us not become weary in doing good, for at the proper time we will reap a harvest if we do not give up" (Galatians 6:9). It's taking the next step when you feel like falling down. Anne Lamott wrote, "Hope begins in the dark, the stubborn hope that if you just show up and try to do the right thing, the dawn will come. You wait and watch and work: You don't give up."[4]

The blessing of the Bible. The Bible is a book of hope. Like going to an ATM to withdraw money, we can go to the Bible to find hope. Daily affirm these twelve reasons you can always have hope in Jesus:

- God is always with you. "Never will I leave you; never will I forsake you" (Hebrews 13:5).
- God loves you as His child. "The Spirit you received brought about your adoption to sonship. And by him we cry, 'Abba, Father.' The Spirit himself testifies with our spirit that we are God's children" (Romans 8:15–16).
- God proved His love at the cross. "He who did not spare his own Son, but gave him up for us all—how will he not also, along with him, graciously give us all things?" (Romans 8:32).
- God's power is available to you. "I can do all this through him who gives me strength" (Philippians 4:13).
- God can exceed your highest expectations. "Now to him who is able to do immeasurably more than all we ask or imagine, according to his power that is at work within us" (Ephesians 3:20).

- God understands you and your problem. "Do not be like them, for your Father knows what you need before you ask him" (Matthew 6:8).

- God promises to supply all your needs. "And my God will meet all your needs according to the riches of his glory in Christ Jesus" (Philippians 4:19).

- God's grace is sufficient for you. "'My grace is sufficient for you, for my power is made perfect in weakness.' Therefore I will boast all the more gladly about my weaknesses, so that Christ's power may rest on me" (2 Corinthians 12:9).

- God works all things together for good. "And we know that in all things God works for the good of those who love him, who have been called according to his purpose" (Romans 8:28).

- God uses trials to produce maturity. "Consider it pure joy, my brothers and sisters, whenever you face trials of many kinds, because you know that the testing of your faith produces perseverance. Let perseverance finish its work so that you may be mature and complete, not lacking anything" (James 1:2–4).

- God uses trials to display our faith. "So that you may become blameless and pure, 'children of God without fault in a warped and crooked generation.' Then you will shine among them like stars in the sky" (Philippians 2:15).

- God's will is good, acceptable, and perfect. "Do not conform to the pattern of this world, but be transformed by the renewing of your mind. Then you will be able to test and approve what God's will is—his good, pleasing and perfect will" (Romans 12:2).[5]

BEYOND THE BOOK

Takeaway: How full is your hope bucket?

Verse to memorize: "May the God of hope fill you with all joy and peace as you trust in him, so that you may overflow with hope by the power of the Holy Spirit" (Romans 15:13).

Question to consider: How full is your hope bucket? Circle the one that applies to you, draw it in the bucket, and date it.

- Empty

- Midway

- Full

Reflections: _____

_____

_____

_____

_____

_____

Prayer: *Lord, my hope bucket is empty. My future seems bleak. Thank You that Your hope bucket is continually overflowing. Please pour Your endless hope into my empty soul. By faith, I choose to believe that one day my hope will rise again. Until then, I choose not to give up, but to press on and take life one day at a time. Amen.*

Application: In another journal, create a safety plan. Outline what you will do and who you will reach out to if you sink into a low mental state.

CHAPTER SEVEN

The Value of Values

He regarded disgrace for the sake of Christ as of greater value than the treasures of Egypt, because he was looking ahead to his reward.

Hebrews 11:26

"Lord, doesn't it seem unfair to you that my sister just sits here while I do all the work? Tell her to come and help me" (Luke 10:40 NLT).

Those are the words of a woman named Martha. She might have looked at her sister, Mary, with her arms crossed and her jaw clenched. She might have loudly sighed and thought, *My sister is so lazy. Why isn't she over here helping me?*

While Martha was busy preparing for Jesus, Mary sat at His feet listening to Him. Mary was focused on *being* with Jesus, while Martha was focused on *doing* for Jesus.

Ironically, Jesus sides with Mary. "My dear Martha, you are worried and upset over all these details! There is only one thing worth being concerned about. Mary has discovered it, and it will not be taken away from her" (Luke 10:41–42 NLT).

What if Martha and Mary represent two modes of being? Those in the "Martha Camp" pride themselves on being busy. Their attitude is, "If you have time to lean, you have time to clean. Don't just stand there, do something." They pride themselves on having a full to-do list.

On the other hand, people in the "Mary Camp" have a different priority. They do not oppose doing for Jesus. Instead, they ensure their doing for Jesus flows out of first being with Jesus. Abiding comes before achieving. Waiting comes before working. Being comes before doing.

Are you more like Mary or Martha?

The Importance of Values

In this story, one of the principles that Jesus teaches Martha about is values. Values clarify priorities and describe what is important to a person. They say that A is more important than B.

Jesus teaches Martha that *being* with Him needs to precede *doing* for Him. Relationship comes before service. Patrick Klingaman drives home the importance of relationships. "What does God value? He wants us to love Him, ourselves (if we don't love ourselves, then loving our neighbor as ourselves has little value), and others with all that we are. That means loving relationships are His priority for us."[1]

Are loving relationships your top priority? Loving God? Loving yourself? Loving others?

Slow Down to Be with Jesus

"Lord, slow me down," was the prayer of W. E. Sangster, a twentieth-century pastor.[2]

Do you need to start praying that prayer? Do you need to slow down to be with Jesus? In *The Ruthless Elimination of Hurry*, John Mark Comer wrote about the danger of busyness. "Corrie ten Boom once said that if the devil can't make you sin, he'll make you busy. There's truth in that. Both sin and busyness have the exact same effect—they cut off your connection to God, to other people, and even to your own soul."[3]

God's Values

One reason sitting at Jesus' feet is so important is that as you do, you will learn His priorities, values, and commands. You can then adopt them as your own. A wise person values what Jesus values.

During the dimness of my depression, my core values, the ones I gleaned from sitting at Jesus' feet, became my lighthouses. They guided me when I didn't know where to turn. My core values became my "why." They directed me when my feelings were telling me to take a wrong turn. Like a sailor lost at sea who looks to the lighthouse for guidance, my values showed me the way when I felt surrounded by darkness.

The Value of Values

Why is it unwise to trust ourselves? Why is it unwise to make your feelings your leader? "Those who trust in themselves are fools, but those who walk in wisdom are kept safe" (Proverbs 28:26).

They can mislead you. Many days over the years, I have awakened and felt anxious or depressed. I didn't feel like doing anything. I didn't feel like pastoring. I felt like lying in bed all day. There were even Sundays when I didn't feel like going to church. On those days, I acknowledged my feelings.

I am feeling depressed. Sad. Anxious. Tired, I tell myself.

Next, I practice something called "Living in the And." This is when I acknowledge my feelings, but instead of allowing them to direct my steps, I choose to subordinate my feelings to God's Word and values. To do this, I practice a principle called "Doing the Opposite." In short, following God's Word and living according to my values often goes against my momentary feelings.

"I feel depressed, *and* I am going to go to church."

"I feel anxious, *and* I am still going to socialize."

"I feel defeated, *and* I am going to minister to that person."

I choose to allow my eternal values to guide me, not my temporary feelings. Do I bat a thousand? No. But that is my goal. My aim is to subordinate my feelings to God's values. This is the essence of personal leadership. Years ago, I read that 50 percent of leadership is leading yourself. At the time, I didn't understand it. I saw leadership more in terms of influencing others than leading myself. Over the years, I have realized the truth of that statement because our greatest leadership tool is our example. The question is not if we are setting an example, but rather, what kind of example we are setting. Your core values will guide you to setting a good example.

Define your core values. I encourage you to carve out time to sit at the feet of Jesus and define your core values by asking questions like these:

- What does a meaningful life look like?
- What is most important to me?
- What would I want said about me at my funeral?
- What does God value?
- How can I make His values mine?

Try to devise a list of five to seven values from your responses. Values like these:

- Faith
- Family
- Health
- Integrity
- Compassion

Imagine if one of your core values was to glorify God. "So whether you eat or drink or whatever you do, do it all for the glory of God" (1 Corinthians 10:31). What if glorifying God was your top goal?

Jonathan Edwards, a pastor during the eighteenth century, wrote a list of resolutions for his life. One of those resolutions was, "Resolved, that I will do whatsoever I think to be most to God's glory . . . never to do any manner of thing, whether in soul or body, less or more, but what tends to the glory of God."[4] God's glory was his utmost aim. Imagine if it became yours! Because of that core value, your prayers might become less about *getting* out of your depression and more about *glorifying* Him in the depression. Imagine if you prayed every day, "Lord, help me to glorify You in this difficult valley. I chose to trust that You will bring me out when it is according to Your will."

Make value-based decisions. After you have clarified your core values, filter your decisions through them. Ask, "Does this decision align with my core values?" If it does, do it. If not, avoid it. This really simplifies the decision-making process. The reason it is so important to make value-based decisions is because you will often end up where your decisions bring you. Ask God to help you choose wisely. Recall His wonderful promise, "I will instruct you and teach you in the way you should go" (Psalm 32:8).

Schedule your core values. After defining our core values, we must, according to Richard Swenson, "place our priorities at the center of our existence and our lives in balanced orbit about these priorities. Placing our lives in a stable, balanced orbit around our core priorities is the first step in achieving a balanced life."[5]

The question is not if you are busy. The real question is, Are you busy doing the essential, eternal things?

Put another way, don't hope to have time for your core values —make time. One of the ways you can do that is by creating margin in your calendar. "Margin is about making space for the things that matter most," wrote Swenson, "while balance is about preserving space for the things that matter most."[6] Are you proactively putting the things that matter most into your schedule, or are you allowing less important things to come before them?

The reason this is important is because when you are depressed, you have limited energy. A wise person chooses to invest their energy in activities that move them toward their core values. Ask yourself, "How can I invest my limited energy in activities that align with my core values?"

Contemplate your core values. Intentionally choose to meditate on your core values. Think about them often. Ponder them regularly because:

> When you intensely and consistently focus on your spiritual values and goals, you increase the blood flow to your frontal lobes and anterior cingulate, which causes the activity in emotional centers of the brain to decrease. Conscious intention is the key, and the more you focus on your inner values, the more you can take charge of your life.[7]

May God communicate to you His lighthouse values as you sit at the feet of Jesus! May you make His values yours.

BEYOND THE BOOK

Takeaway: Make values-based decisions, not feeling-led ones.

Verse to memorize: "He regarded disgrace for the sake of Christ as of greater value than the treasures of Egypt, because he was looking ahead to his reward" (Hebrews 11:26).

Question to consider: Imagine that your biography was published in the local newspaper. What would you want your family, friends, and coworkers to say about you? From this exercise, discern your top five to seven values.

Reflections: _____

_____

_____

_____

_____

Prayer: *Lord, life is busy. Sometimes I get so busy doing activities that I neglect being with You. Please help me prioritize being with You over doing things for You. Please clarify what is truly important as I sit at Your feet and listen to Your voice. After I define my values, please give me the moral muscle to follow them, subordinating my temporary feelings to Your eternal values. I appreciate Your grace when I fall short. By faith, today, I choose to be value-led over feeling-led. Amen.*

Application: Values Audit: Write out what you did today. Next to each item on the list, mark which value it aligns with. Then ponder your list and ask, Which values are represented well? Which values need more representation?

CHAPTER EIGHT

The Call of Compassion

The LORD is compassionate and gracious, slow to anger, abounding in love.

Psalm 103:8

In 1950, Mother Teresa established the Missionaries of Charity, a ministry that would care for the dying and destitute in Calcutta, India. Sacrificially, she modeled love and service to people experiencing poverty. Her compassion caught the world's attention, and she won the Nobel Peace Prize in 1979. Her motto was, "It is not how much we do, but how much love we put into what we do."[1]

Mother Theresa was short in stature but large in influence. One of the traits that caused her to make such an impact was her contagious smile. It could light up a room. Because of her infectious smile, it would be easy to assume she was always happy.

She wasn't.

Throughout 1946 and 1947, Mother Teresa experienced a profound union with Christ. But soon after she left the convent and began her work among the destitute and dying on the street, the visions and locutions ceased, and she experienced a spiritual darkness that would remain with her until her death.[2]

And Mother Teresa tells us:

I am told God loves me—and yet the reality of darkness and cold-ness and emptiness is so great that nothing touches my soul. Before the work started, there was so much union, love, faith, trust, prayer, and sacrifice. Did I make a mistake in surrendering blindly to the Call of the Sacred Heart?[3]

Behind Mother Teresa's vibrant smile and sacrificial service was deep depression. Outwardly she showed love and compassion to others, while inwardly she felt dark and depressed. Perhaps there is a lesson here. What if her example illustrates what I call the compassion cure? What if showing love and compassion to others will lift us to a higher level of mental well-being?

The Definition of Compassion

According to the Bible, *compassion* means "to have mercy, to feel sympathy and to have pity."[4] Compassion is showing mercy and empathy toward others. Jesus modeled compassion. "When he saw the crowds, he had compassion on them, because they were harassed and helpless, like sheep without a shepherd" (Matthew 9:36). God is compassionate. "The LORD is compassionate and gracious, slow to anger, abounding in love" (Psalm 103:8).

The Daily Dose of Compassion

Discouraged and depressed, Jeremiah, the weeping prophet, bares his soul to God.

Cursed be the day I was born! May the day my mother bore me not be blessed! Cursed be the man who brought my father the news, who made him very glad, saying, "A child is born to you—a son!"

. . . Why did I ever come out of the womb to see trouble and sorrow and to end my days in shame?

Jeremiah 20:14–18

Living such a hard life, he does not consider his birth a blessing—just the opposite. In the second book Jeremiah wrote, Lamentations, he shares a wonderful reason to have hope. "Because of the LORD's great love we are not consumed, for his compassions never fail. They are new every morning; great is your faithfulness" (Lamentations 3:22–23).

God's love and compassion are new every morning. Every day is a new opportunity to experience God's mercy and grace. What if you anticipated the compassion of God as your eyes opened in the morning? Visualize awakening every morning expecting God's compassion in the same way you anticipate drinking your morning coffee. Before you get out of bed, picture praying, "Lord, thank You that a fresh pot of compassion is awaiting me," as you smell the toasty, slightly burnt fragrance from the coffee pot.

The Benefits of Compassion

Since God is compassionate, we would be wise to follow His example. As we do, we will discover mental health benefits. In their book *Compassionate Leadership,* Engstrom and Cedar write that Dr. Karl Menninger, founder of the famed Menninger Clinic, discovered "that people who give of themselves in service to others are the happiest and healthiest."[5]

What if compassion is a hidden pathway to joy? What if compassionate action is the doorway to inner satisfaction? "Those who refresh others will themselves be refreshed" (Proverbs 11:25 NLT).

Are you open to trying the compassion cure? What if your attitude was, "No matter what I do or where I am, I can love and be of service to others."[6]

As you try the compassionate cure, you will find that it is in lifting others that you rise. In blessing others, you are blessed. In helping others, you are helped.

Find Someone to Help

"Doctor, I feel depressed," the patient said as he sat in the hospital room. He had sad eyes, a long face, and a defeated demeanor. The doctor took notes on a clipboard and thought about his prescription.

"I want you to leave your apartment daily and look for someone to help. Do this once a day and report back to me in a week."

The patient silently protested, thinking, *Do what? I am having a hard enough time making it through the day, and you want me to help others?* He was, however, desperate enough to give it a try.

"Who can I help today?" the man declared every day as he left his house. As he began to focus on helping others, the strangest thing happened—he started to feel better.

"How did it go?" asked the doctor at their next meeting.

The man smiled. "I feel so much better. I can't believe how much better I feel."

This troubled man found out that by helping others, he felt helped. John Keble said, "When you find yourself . . . overpowered as it were by melancholy, the best way is to go out, and do something kind."[7]

The Practice of Self-Compassion

I know people who talk to themselves in ways they would never talk to others . . . even their worst enemy. They are compassionate to others and condemning toward themselves.

This is wrong!

"Love your neighbor *as yourself*," said Jesus (Matthew 22:39, emphasis added). We are not just to show compassion to others but to show compassion to ourselves. Use the compassionate cure on yourself. When you are experiencing a difficult day, talk to yourself in a compassionate tone, saying, "I feel depressed today. I know others are in the same boat as me. I will make it because I have the support of God, my loving family, and my friends. I will focus on doing the next right thing."

The Discovery of Compassion

One of my regular practices is writing handwritten notes to people to encourage or thank them. I remember visiting one of the members of our church and seeing a note I had written to them hanging on their fridge. I had written it about six months prior.

People have told me how meaningful these notes are to them. It breathes life into their spirits; however, what they don't realize is that it also breathes life into my spirit. As a young pastor, I wrote these notes to show people I cared about them. As I did this, I noticed something unexpected—I felt encouraged. As I wrote those notes of appreciation, I felt grateful. In short, when I blessed others, I felt blessed. It's the compassion cure.

How can you be a blessing to someone today? You say, "But Steve, I am so depressed. All I want to do is stay under the covers and cry." I understand. I have been there. What if Mother Teresa became your example? What if you added compassion to your list of values and declared, "I feel depressed *and* I am going to show love and compassion to others."

Who can you show compassion to today? Don't forget to share your compassion to the person in the mirror!

─────────────── **BEYOND THE BOOK** ───────────────

Takeaway: Today I will try the compassion cure, knowing that it is in lifting others, I rise, in blessing others, I am blessed, and in helping others, I am helped.

Verse to memorize: "The Lord is compassionate and gracious, slow to anger, abounding in love" (Psalm 103:8).

Question to consider: What keeps me from showing compassion to those around me?

Reflections:

_____

_____

_____

_____

_____

Prayer: *Lord, I struggle with selfishness. I spend way too much time thinking about my needs, desires, and wants. Please flip a switch in me so that I will focus less on my needs and more on the needs of others. Please fill my heart with compassion so that I can share it with those I meet today. Open my eyes to see those You have brought into my life today who need Your help. Please bring life to my spirit as I practice the compassion cure. Amen.*

Application: Make a list of five people and what you plan to do to meet their needs. When you are done, write the date in the "done" box.

Name	How I plan to meet their needs?	Done
My neighbor Bill	*Shovel his driveway*	*1/21/25*

The Spiritual Key

Name	How I plan to meet their needs?	Done

PART TWO

The Mental Key

Love the Lord your God . . . with all your mind.

Mark 12:30

CHAPTER NINE

The Gift of Gratitude

Give thanks in all circumstances; for this is God's will for you in Christ Jesus.

1 Thessalonians 5:18

In the spring of 1934, Harold Abbott of Webb City, Missouri, was walking down the road with his tail between his legs. He felt defeated. His grocery store had closed the previous Saturday, and he had accumulated so much debt that would take him seven years to repay. "I walked like a beaten man. I had lost all my fight and faith," he said.

But then something happened that drastically changed his life. He came upon a man on the street who had no legs. He was sitting on a wooden base with wheels from roller skates, and that is how he got around.

"Good morning, sir. It is a fine morning, isn't it?" said the man with no legs.

Harold was touched to the heart and scolded himself. *Here is a man who has no legs yet is jolly. I have both legs and am not.* He determined that day to focus on appreciating what he had in life instead of focusing on what he did not have. He posted a saying on his bathroom mirror that he read every morning:

I had the blues because I had no shoes,
Until upon the street, I met a man who had no feet.[1]

After telling that story in his book, *How to Stop Worrying and Start Living,* Dale Carnegie asks:

Would you sell both your eyes for a billion dollars? What would you take for your two legs? Your hands? Your hearing? Your children? Your family? Add up your assets, and you will find that that you won't sell what you have for all the gold ever amassed by the Rockefellers, the Fords and the Morgans combined.[2]

The story illustrates one of my favorite mental health tools: gratitude. Gratitude is the attitude of thankfulness. It's counting your blessings. It's appreciating the goodness of God in your life.

It's important to develop a thankful spirit because God's will for you is to be thankful—not *for* all situations but *in* all situations. "Give thanks in all circumstances; for this is God's will for you in Christ Jesus" (1 Thessalonians 5:18). A good example of this was David.

The Gratitude of David

David faced many challenges in his life, yet he always seemed to put his ultimate hope in God. In Psalm 16, David shares five reasons he was grateful to God:

God was his refuge. "Keep me safe, my God, for in you I take refuge" (Psalm 16:1). In the Bible, a refuge is a safe place of protection or shelter. God was David's refuge. His safe place. He went to God for safety and security when he felt unsafe and uncertain. We can do the same. Like David, we can go through scary seasons. Perhaps you are in one of those seasons right now. May you follow David's example and turn to God as your refuge. "I will say of the LORD, 'He is my refuge and my fortress, my God, in whom I trust'" (Psalm 91:2).

God is a good provider. "LORD, you alone are my portion and my cup; you make my lot secure" (Psalm 16:5).

David declares that God is his portion and cup. Portion refers to inheritance, and cup refers to blessings. God was his blessed inheritance. In addition, he mentions that God makes his lot secure. The word *lot* recalls the time when God gave the gift of Canaan to Israel and divided it by lots. Each family got the lot God gave them.

One of the ways we can be more grateful is to be content with our lot. Are you content with the lot God has given you? Or are you jealous of the lot He has given someone else?

The enemy of contentment is envy. Instead of appreciating what you have, envy wants what others have. It is desiring what is not yours. It's a sin. "You shall not covet your neighbor's house. You shall not covet your neighbor's wife, or his male or female servant, his ox or donkey, or anything that belongs to your neighbor" (Exodus 20:17).

Since envy is a sin, and sin robs us of the abundant life God has for us, we need to avoid it at all costs. One of the best ways to do that is to replace an envious heart with a grateful one.

Gratitude is the antidote of envy.

Envy and gratitude are like oil and water. They are incompatible. If you intentionally practice gratitude, you will find the envy driven out of your spirit. A practical way to do that is by practicing the habit of "thankful prayer," which is spending half your prayer time thanking God for the blessings you already have, and the other half asking for more blessings.

God is a good counselor. "I will praise the LORD, who counsels me; even at night my heart instructs me" (Psalm 16:7). David saw God as his counselor, therapist, comforter, and helper. He learned to share his burdens with the Lord and receive His help. We can do the same thing. We can cast our cares on the Holy Spirit, whom the Bible calls our Advocate.

> And I will ask the Father, and he will give you another advocate to help you and be with you forever—the Spirit of truth. The world cannot accept him, because it neither sees him nor knows him. But you know him, for he lives with you and will be in you.
>
> John 14:16–17

Other translations of the Bible refer to the Advocate as the Comforter. He will counsel us, support us, and help us.

God is near. "I keep my eyes always on the LORD. With him at my right hand, I will not be shaken" (Psalm 16:8).

David contemplated the closeness of God. He kept his eye on the Lord. As he did, he grew in confidence. We can follow his example. As followers of Jesus, we have the Holy Spirit living within us. He is also known as the Comforter, Advocate, or Helper. He comes alongside us and supports us. "My Presence will go with you, and I will give you rest" (Exodus 33:14).

God is your eternal hope. "Because you will not abandon me to the realm of the dead, nor will you let your faithful one see decay. You make known to me the path of life; you will fill me with joy in your presence, with eternal pleasures at your right hand" (Psalm 16:10–11).

David's optimism came from knowing that the end of this life is not the end. Our body may die, but our spirit lives on in eternity with Christ, if we are a believer. "Someday you will read or hear that Billy Graham is dead. Don't you believe a word of it. I shall be more alive than I am now. I will have just changed my address."[3]

"Surely your goodness and love will follow me all the days of my life, and I will dwell in the house of the LORD forever" (Psalm 23:6).

Imagine cultivating a daily habit of dwelling on the goodness of God. Imagine if we thought less about the world's imperfections and more about God's perfections.

Since gratitude is so important to our overall mental well-being, I want to close by sharing with you two other practical ways to develop a thankful spirit.

The Other Side of the Coin

A coin has two sides—heads and tails. Most situations also have positive aspects and negative ones. In this exercise, you acknowledge both. If you are wrestling with depression, write down the negative aspects:

- Fatigue
- A lack of zest for living
- Loneliness

Okay. That is one side of the coin. What about the other side? Make a list of the positive things about depression:

- It causes me to depend on God more.
- It gives me greater empathy for those who are struggling with depression.
- Depression is my "credentials" for helping others who are depressed.

This exercise shows us that most situations are not all bad or are all good, but they are usually a combination of both.

The Bookends of Gratitude

Picture a row of books with bookends on both sides. The bookends start and end the rows of books. The bookend of gratitude exercise is the habit of starting and ending your day with gratitude. Before you get out of bed, think about five things you are grateful for. Tell God about them. In addition, before you go to bed, make another gratitude list.

May you be grateful in God! May you recognize the abundance you already have in Him.

BEYOND THE BOOK

Takeaway: Gratitude is the attitude of thankfulness.

Verse to memorize: "Give thanks in all circumstances; for this is God's will for you in Christ Jesus" (1 Thessalonians 5:18).

Question to consider: How have you experienced the goodness of God in your life?

Reflections: _____

_____

_____

_____

_____

_____

Prayer: *Lord Jesus, I live in a materialistic, greedy culture. At times, I have been infected with this greed virus that leads to envy and comparison. As a result, I often desire more and more instead of thanking You for what I already have. Please free me from this trap. Help me to see the abundance I already have in You and in my loved ones. By faith, I chose to develop the habit of thankfulness today. Amen.*

Application: Bookend your day with gratitude. Make a gratitude list in the morning and before you go to bed. Here are some blessings you may want to be thankful for:

- Spiritual blessings
- Material blessings
- Physical blessings
- Relational blessings
- Blessings you are believing God for
- Blessings you are not aware of

CHAPTER TEN

The Antidote to Anxiety

Cast all your anxiety on him because he cares for you.

1 Peter 5:7

A fictional story is told about a man who came face-to-face with Death one day.

Alarmed, he asked, "What are you up to?"

"I'm going to take one hundred people."

"That's horrible!"

"That's the way it is. That's what I do."

Quickly, the man ran to warn everyone he could about Death's plan. "Death is on the loose. He is going to take one hundred people. Be careful." As evening fell, he met Death again. Hearing that a thousand people had died that day, he felt lied to.

"You told me you were going to take one hundred people. Why did one thousand people die?"

"I kept my word. I only took one hundred people. *Worry took the others.*"

What Is Worry?

The author of the book of Hebrews defines faith: "Now faith is the substance of things hoped for, the evidence of things not seen" (Hebrews 11:1 NKJV). Worry is the opposite of faith. "It's the substance of things dreaded, with the evidence not yet seen."[1]

Worry is anticipating Satan's worst instead of God's best.

It has dire consequences. The Hebrew word for *worry* means "division" or "separation into parts."

Worry leads to an internal tug-of-war pulling your insides apart. It scatters your mind and divides your soul. Consequently, "When we leave anxiety unchecked, the thinking part of our brain (the neocortex) loses its effectiveness. When that happens, leadership and relationships suffer."[2]

Knowing the destructive nature of worry, Jesus commands us to avoid it. "That is why I tell you not to worry about everyday life—whether you have enough food and drink, or enough clothes to wear. Isn't life more than food, and your body more than clothing?" (Matthew 6:25 NLT). Personally, this is one of the most challenging commands in the Bible for me to obey. I am a recovering worrywart. It comforts me to know that Paul wrestled with anxiety, too. "Therefore I am all the more eager to send him, so that when you see him again you may be glad and *I may have less anxiety*" (Philippians 2:28, emphasis added).

If you are worried, here are some reminders to help you stop fretting and trust God.

Worrying is a waste of time. "Can all your worries add a single moment to your life?" (Matthew 6:27 NLT). Jesus encourages us to think logically. Does worry add to your life? No. If anything, it steals your life. Reflecting on my life, I've wasted so many precious moments worrying. One of my deepest regrets are the times "Mr. Anxiety" stole from my family, especially from my kids when they were young. Regretfully, I was often so wrapped up in my anxious thoughts that I was not fully engaged. I can relate to the words of Dr. Graham in the movie *Field of Dreams*. "We just don't recognize the most significant moments of our lives while they're happening. Back then, I thought, 'Well, there'll be other days.' I didn't realize that that was the only day."[3]

Worrying is a costly sin!

Moreover, after all these years of worrying, I believe it is a waste of time. Most of my worries have never come true. A study at Penn State confirms the uselessness of worry. In this study, participants recorded their worries for ten days. The participants even received text messages reminding them to document their fears. Then, over the next thirty days, these worriers watched to see if their worries had come true. Their findings?

> A whopping 91 percent of worries were false alarms. And of the remaining 9 percent of worries that did come true, the outcome was better than expected about a third of the time. For about one in four participants, exactly zero of their worries materialized.[4]

Worry is living in the future, not the present. "So don't worry about tomorrow, for tomorrow will bring its own worries. Today's trouble is enough for today" (Matthew 6:34 NLT). Jesus teaches us to live in "day-tight compartments"[5]—to set tight boundaries around our thoughts, not allowing them to wander beyond the present moment. When they cross today's line, we need to take them by the arm and lead them back to the precious present. "It has taken me a long time to realize that my only job is to work at the tasks God has given me to do today," wrote Patrick Klingaman. "Worrying about what needs to be done tomorrow—or what unforeseen event might happen tomorrow—is not my job."[6]

Do your job; trust God to do His!

One of the best ways to live in the present is to learn to focus your mind on the here and now. In his helpful book, *The Mayo Clinic Gude to Stress-Free Living*, Dr. Amit Sood writes about the two modes of your brain: default and focused.[7] The default mode, also called mind wandering, is when your mind is on autopilot and goes with the psychological flow. In the default mode, your mind will move toward threat, pleasure, and novelty; however, its first choice is a threat.

A wandering mind tends to end up in the land of worry!

On the other hand, the focused mode is fully engaged in what you are presently doing. If you are driving home from work, your mind is fully engaged in driving, paying attention to the road, the other drivers, and the conditions of the road. Dr. Sood has found that we are happiest in a focused mindset.

Like a marksman who practices focusing his gun, I encourage you to learn to focus your mind with laser-like intensity on the present moment. Become thoroughly engrossed in the present. Ask yourself, "What do I see? Smell? Taste? Feel? Hear?"

On his podcast, *Boundaries and Me,* Christian psychologist and bestselling author Dr. Henry Cloud recommends a practice called "Feel, Ignore, Engage,"[8] to overcome anxiety. He recommends doing these three steps in chronological order.

Feel. Even though it seems counterintuitive, trying to get rid of a feeling is not wise. When it comes to the nature of feelings, what you resist persists. Instead of trying to get rid of it, feel it.

Ignore. Next, Dr. Cloud teaches us to ignore our negative mental chatter. Say something like, "I noticed that my mind had a negative thought." Don't try to change your nervous thoughts; ignore them.

Engage. Focus your mind on the task at hand. As you chop the wood, notice how the axe feels in your hands. Hear the thud of it hitting the log. See the birds singing in the forest. *The Message* translation of Matthew 6:34 says, "Give your entire attention to what God is doing right now." As you do this, the wave of anxiety will pass.

Worry shows a lack of trust in God. "That is why I tell you not to worry about everyday life—whether you have enough food and drink, or enough clothes to wear. Isn't life more than food, and your body more than clothing?" (Matthew 6:25 NLT). Right after this verse, Jesus points to some flying birds. "Look at the birds" (Matthew 6:26). Just as God provides for the birds, He will provide for us.

The antidote to fear is faith. As we learn to rest in God's fatherly care, the cares of this life melt away. Steve Cuss, in *Managing Leadership Anxiety,* writes:

> The goal of managing anxiety is not simply for relief, it is to connect more fully with God and to raise awareness of what God is

doing. Anxiety blocks our awareness of God because it takes our subconscious attention. This means that anxiety can be an early detection system that we're depending on something other than God for our well-being.[9]

BEYOND THE BOOK

Takeaway: Worry is anticipating Satan's worst instead of God's best.

Verse to memorize: "Do not be anxious about anything, but in every situation, by prayer and petition, with thanksgiving, present your requests to God. And the peace of God, which transcends all understanding, will guard your hearts and your minds in Christ Jesus" (Philippians 4:6–7).

Question to consider: For your reflection today, calculate the "validity quotient"[10] of your worry. Make a list of all the things you have worried about. Next, calculate how many of them have come true. That is your validity quotient.

Reflections: _____

_____

_____

_____

_____

Prayer: *Lord Jesus, I acknowledge my inner anxiety. I admit that I worry too much and pray too little. Help me reverse that sequence. As I choose to worship instead of worry, please move me from fear to faith, pressure to peace, and anxiety to serenity.*

By faith, I choose to embrace Your peace, which surpasses all understanding. Amen.

Application: Set aside time today to practice being in the focused mode. Train your brain to notice details. Use your five senses to immerse yourself fully in the precious present.

CHAPTER ELEVEN

The Training of Thoughts

My thoughts trouble me and I am distraught.

Psalm 55:2

"I am wrestling with fear," he said, with tears in his eyes. I could hear the fear and uncertainty in his voice as he spoke about his wife who was lying unconscious on a hospital bed. A nurse was in the corner carefully monitoring her.

"I know I should have faith, but I am catastrophizing. What if she doesn't make it? What if I lose her? What would I do without her?"

I listened intently and showed empathy.

"She is the anchor of our family," he replied, putting his head in his hands. "I don't know what I would do without her." As he talked, I prayed for him. *Lord, please help him. Give him strength.*

Shaking his head in disgust, he said, "I have these scary, intrusive thoughts. I know I should trust God. But I don't know what to do with these thoughts." Then he said something that has stuck with me.

"These thoughts are causing me to go to a dark place."

Can you relate? Are your thoughts causing you to go to a dark place? Are they sending you into a downward spiral of anxiety and fear?

The Power of Our Thoughts

Perhaps you are downplaying the importance of your thoughts. *They are just a few harmless thoughts. What's the big deal?* you think.

Wrong!

Our thoughts are incredibly powerful. They are precursors to our feelings and actions. If you want to change your behaviors and feelings, you must first change your thoughts. "For as he thinketh in his heart, so is he" (Proverbs 23:7 KJV)

Moreover, our psychology affects our biology. "Your thoughts, too, can change your biochemistry. That's right; what you are thinking right now can actually change the chemical composition of your brain cells and the rest of your central nervous system."[1] The meditations of your mind can change the chemicals of your brain! Since our thoughts are so powerful, perhaps we should pray this Celtic prayer daily: "God be in my head."[2]

The power of our thoughts should not surprise us because the Bible teaches, "Be transformed by the renewing of your mind" (Romans 12:2). Like a caterpillar being transformed into a butterfly, our lives are metamorphosed as we renew our mind with God's Word.

In this chapter, I want to share with you thought strategies that can help you experience greater levels of mental well-being.

Take Your Thoughts Captive

Paul reminds us that the nature of true reality is that we are in a spiritual battle.

The weapons we fight with are not the weapons of the world. On the contrary, they have divine power to demolish strongholds. We demolish arguments and every pretension that sets itself up against the knowledge of God, and we take captive every thought to make it obedient to Christ.

2 Corinthians 10:4–5

Since it is a spiritual battle, our weapons are not natural ones—spears, swords, or shields. They are spiritual—prayer, words, and worship. In this battle, wrong thinking can lead to strongholds of the mind. The antidote is to take every thought captive. In other words, when a thought passes through your mind, challenge it by asking, "Does this thought align with God's Word?" Here are seven thoughts to be on guard for:

Seven Toxic Thought Patterns

As I go over the list, remember that "you can't control the train of thoughts coming your way, but you can decide whether or not you want to get on the train."[3]

Pessimistic forecast. *The bottom is going to fall out. Doom and gloom are on the horizon.* Thoughts like this fall into the category of negative predictions. Your mind predicts that your future is bleak. When this happens, you need to remind yourself that no one knows the future but God. Tell yourself, "My future is in your hands" (Psalm 31:15 NLT).

Undervaluing your resilience in Christ. *If such and such happens, I won't be able to endure it.* Thoughts like this can cause you to question God's ability to get you through a trial or difficulty. Remind yourself of God's faithfulness in the past. The same God who got you through yesterday's storms will get you through the storms of today . . . and tomorrow.

Negative assessment. Imagine that a loved one doesn't respond to your text right away. *They are mad at me. They don't want anything to do with me,* you think. This is an example of negative appraisal. It is evaluating things in a negative light.

When you find yourself appraising someone's action in a negative light, practice the principle of "when in doubt, check it out."

Tell the person, "My perception is that you didn't return my text because you are upset with me. Is that accurate?"

Another helpful tool is to come up with five alternative interpretations of an event. Imagine, for example, that you have a controlling, micromanaging boss. *This is horrible. They are ruining my life,* you think. What are five different ways you could interpret their actions?

1. My boss is giving me an education of what *not* to do.
2. My boss is giving me an opportunity to love my enemies.
3. My boss is giving me an opportunity to get my identity from Jesus, not my job.
4. My boss is giving me an opportunity to practice brave communication as I tell my boss how they are hurting me.
5. My boss is giving me an opportunity to pray for my enemies.

Brooding over. Imagine a cow chewing their cud, mulling it over and over. In a similar way, we can practice negative rumination, mulling over a negative thought. When this happens, push the pause button and see it as a reminder to practice biblical mediation. Rumination is worry; biblical meditation is worship. "I will consider all your works and meditate on all your mighty deeds" (Psalm 77:12).

All-or-nothing thinking. All-or-nothing thinking is extreme thinking. It's seeing people as all good or all bad. The truth is that, as Christians, we are a combination of saint and sinner. Most situations are also not all good or all bad.

Overgeneralization. Overgeneralization is when you apply a specific incident to all incidents. It's when you take the behaviors of a particular person and project them onto others. *Since one person hurt me, all people will hurt me,* you think. The truth is that some people will hurt you, but others will love you. The remedy for overgeneralization is to remember that specific is terrific. Perhaps, for example, you go home every night thinking, *I am a* *bad manager.* Is that the truth? Probably not. A more accurate assessment might be, *I am gifted in certain parts of managing—listening, being calm under pressure, and being approachable. I need to work on other areas, such as holding people accountable, dealing with conflict, and giving more direct guidance.*

Personalizing. Personalizing is when you interpret the actions of others as a reflection of you and not them. It's when you see their choices and words as an indictment against you. *My spouse left because I was a lousy spouse*, you think.

Wrong!

Their behavior reflects them, not you. "So then, each of us will give an account of ourselves to God" (Romans 14:12). Note that we are not accountable for other people's actions—only for our own.

Thought management. Before planting Community Celebration Church, I was the manager of Men's Wearhouse, a men's clothing store. My duties were to manage the staff and inventory and to provide excellent customer service. As the manager, I could determine who was allowed to be in our store and who needed to leave. If, for example, someone was toxic to our team, I could ask them to leave.

Similarly, you are the manager of your mind. What thoughts are you allowing to dwell in your mind? When a belligerent, toxic though enters your mind, take it captive in Christ and cast it out. Intentionally think God's thoughts, which are found in His Word.

BEYOND THE BOOK

Takeaway: You are a thought manager.

Verse to memorize: "May these words of my mouth and this meditation of my heart be pleasing in your sight, LORD, my Rock and my Redeemer" (Psalm 19:14).

Question to consider: Which of the seven toxic thought patterns in this chapter do you wrestle with?

Y or N: Pessimistic forecast

Y or N: Undervaluing your resilience in Christ

Y or N: Negative assessment

Y or N: Brooding over

Y or N: All-or-nothing thinking

Y or N: Overgeneralization

Y or N: Personalizing

Reflections: ....

....

....

....

....

....

Prayer: *Lord, sometimes I feel as though my thoughts are out of control. I need Your help managing them. Help me be aware of toxic thoughts so that I can use "thought judo" and leverage them to think Your thoughts. By faith, I chose to become a conscientious thought manager, kicking toxic thoughts out and inviting nourishing thoughts into the garden of my mind.*

Application: Practice the five alternative interpretations exercise. Write out the answers to these questions in a journal.[4]

- What happened?
- How are you interpreting it?
- What are five different ways you could interpret it?
- Which interpretation aligns with God's truth?

CHAPTER TWELVE

The Function of Feelings

Jesus was indignant.

Mark 1:41

In February of 2020, Tammy and I drove twelve hours in a blizzard to attend a marriage retreat in Michigan. *It's as if Satan doesn't want us to go*, I thought as I passed our church, which was closed that morning because of bad weather. Our church was ten minutes from my house. The drive to the retreat was twelve hours. Battling the snow-laden roads, bone-chilling wind, and icy roads made for a long day. By the grace of God, we arrived at a beautiful log house around eight that night.

Before we left for the retreat, Tammy told me that she didn't think our marriage would last.

"I don't even know why I am going to the retreat. I am done."

"There are no expectations," I said. "Let's just go and see what happens." She agreed to go. As we brought our suitcases to our room, I thought, *This retreat is like a Hail Mary pass in football. We need a miracle.*

The following day, as we waited to join eight other struggling couples for group counseling, I found a moment of peace staring at the flickering fire in the fireplace. As the session started, the leaders of the retreat had the couples go around and share why they were there. As they did, I found hope in the fact that we were not alone in our struggles. In fact, there was another clergy couple in the group.

I filled a whole notebook with the lessons I learned at that retreat.[1] One lesson, however, stands above the rest. When one of the leaders shared the following truth, I felt as if I had an epiphany.

"Communication is like an iceberg," she said, as she drew an iceberg on the white board. "Ten percent of an iceberg is above water. In communication, that is akin to the content and logic of a conversation. Many couples are good at connecting at this level—the ten percent above the water level." Next, she pointed to the largest part of the iceberg, the part that is underwater.

"Ninety percent of an iceberg is below the water. This is akin to the feelings, fears, and desires of communication. Many couples do not know how to connect on this below the surface level."

Bingo. That is us, I thought.

At that moment, I realized that Tammy and I were connecting with our heads but not our hearts. We were connecting on a practical level but not an emotional level. As the week went on, I realized the reason I had difficulty connecting with her on an emotional level was because I had an erroneous view of feelings. David's example brought me clarity.

David's Example

David shares his raw emotions with God.

> How long, LORD? Will you forget me forever? How long will you hide your face from me? How long must I wrestle with my thoughts and day after day have sorrow in my heart? How long will my enemy triumph over me?"
>
> Psalm 13:1–2

He doesn't try to sugarcoat those thoughts. "I have sorrow in my heart," he writes. Psalm 13 fits into a category of psalms called psalms of lament. One-third of all the psalms fit into this category. Mark Vroegop, in *Dark Clouds, Deep Mercy* defines lament as "the honest cry of a hurting heart wrestling with the paradox of pain and the promise of God's goodness."[2]

Since there are so many of these psalms of lament, we can deduce that God wants us to be honest with Him. Rather than numbing, stuffing, or ignoring our feelings, He wants us to express them openly to Him. Gary Neal Hansen, in *Kneeling with Giants,* agrees:

> The psalms show us our own experience as in a mirror, and then they put a megaphone in our hand so we can speak to God about that experience. This is what Calvin meant when he famously called the psalms an anatomy book of the human soul. In the psalms he saw overflowing joy, rapturous praise, awe and reverence, peaceful stillness, but he also saw boastful pride, brokenhearted depression, vindictive rage and lonely abandonment. As biblical prayers, the psalms invite us to include this full range in our own prayers.[3]

The Truth About Feelings

To grow in emotional intelligence, we must learn the truth about feelings. First, there are six categories of feelings:[4]

- Happiness
- Sadness
- Anger
- Fear
- Disgust
- Surprise

What is the purpose of our feelings? Why did God give us feelings? "Think of your emotions as God's information system," writes Gary Smalley. "They inform you about your needs and your deepest beliefs. When you feel a strong emotion—fear, let's say, or grief—your body is trying to tell you something important."[5]

Said another way, feelings are like the dashboard lights on your car. They're trying to communicate to you something about your soul. Are you listening? A great question to ask yourself is, "What are my feelings trying to communicate to me?"

The Source of Our Feelings

As human beings, we are emotional beings. Our emotions come from being made in the image of God.

> We often forget that God has emotions, too. He feels things very deeply. The Bible tells us that God grieves, gets jealous and angry, and feels compassion, pity, sorrow, and sympathy as well as happiness, gladness, and satisfaction. God loves, delights, gets pleasure, rejoices, enjoys, and even laughs.[6]

What Do I Do with My Feelings?

There are a few things I suggest that we do after we recognize the source and strength of our emotions.

Feel your feelings. I believed that a good Christian should not feel anger, bitterness, anxiety, sadness, or discouragement. As a result of this faulty belief, I learned to stuff, ignore, and suppress my feelings. This was unwise because, "What we resist persists. Feelings we attempt to suppress simply go on longer, and often turn into chronic emotional disorders."[7]

Suppressing our feelings is akin to pushing a beach ball down into the water. We stuff it down, down, and down only to have it explode out of the water. Instead of suppressing our feelings, we should express them in a healthy way. Remember that our feelings are like a cloud in the sky that will eventually pass by us. Feel your feelings in faith and ask God to help you act according to His Word, not your mood.

Name it, tame it. Develop the habit of naming your emotions. When you sense you are angry, say to yourself, "I am feeling angry." By naming your uncomfortable feelings, you bring them out of the darkness and into the light. As a result, they lose their power over you.

Examine your self-talk. Motivational speaker Brian Tracy wrote that "95% of your emotions are determined by the way you talk to yourself."[8] If you desire invigorating feelings, talk to yourself in a nurturing way. Train yourself to talk to yourself with the utmost love and respect.

A great example of healthy self-talk is, "Why, my soul, are you downcast? Why so disturbed within me? Put your hope in God, for I will yet praise him, my Savior and my God" (Psalm 42:5). Do you see how the psalmist is questioning his discouragement and focusing his mind on the goodness of God?

How do you talk to the person in the mirror? Learn to monitor your self-talk, because as Martin Seligman, author of *Learned Optimism* writes, "Anytime you find yourself down or anxious or angry, ask what you're saying to yourself."[9]

Venting to God

Earlier in this chapter, I shared about the psalms of lament, which teach us to openly express our pain to God. Would you consider praying a prayer of lament the next time you are struggling? It has four parts to it:

- Chose to turn toward God.
- Openly express your pain and emotions to God.
- Ask for His help.
- Choose to trust Him no matter how you feel.[10]

During my 2002 storm, a prayer of lament might have looked like this:

Lord, I choose to turn to You in this difficult season. I feel like quitting the ministry and giving up. Please help me see my situation from Your perspective. Help me learn the lessons in this storm You intend for me to learn. Help me to keep on keeping on. By faith, I choose to trust that You will bring good out of this difficult time. I cannot see it, but I choose to believe it. I choose to trust You even though I don't understand what You are up to. In the strong name of Jesus, Amen.

The Drive Home

We came to the retreat in a blizzard, internally and externally. Our marriage had grown cold and distant. God did a great work in our hearts during that week in the cabin. As we made the long drive back to Minnesota, Tammy said, "Let's start dating again."

Praise the Lord!

BEYOND THE BOOK

Takeaway: Jesus is your leader, not your feelings. Feel your feelings, but don't blindly follow them—follow Jesus!

Verse to memorize: "Jesus was indignant" (Mark 1:41).

Questions to consider: What is my relationship to my feelings? Do I view them in a healthy, biblical way? Why or why not?

Reflections: _____

_____

_____

_____

_____

Prayer: *Lord Jesus, thank You for making me in Your image. Just as You have feelings, so do I. Help me to have a proper relationship with my feelings, not deifying or demonizing them but seeing them as an information system. By faith, I choose to acknowledge my feelings without being led by them. I choose to be led by Your Spirit and Word instead. Amen.*

Application: In your journal, write out a prayer of lament, using all four of the elements mentioned above.

CHAPTER THIRTEEN

The Joy of Journaling

Then the LORD said to Moses, "Write this on a scroll as something to be remembered."

Exodus 17:14

In the eighteenth century, a missionary named David Brainerd kept a journal of his walk with God and his passion for reaching God's lost children. Reading those journals has inspired countless Christians throughout history to live a Christlike life.

The impact of Brainerd's life on the evangelical missionary vision and Christian enterprise generally has been invaluable. Consider the galaxy of worthy names directly involved in missions who have acknowledged a great debt to reading Brainerd's life; John Wesley, Francis Asbury, William Carey, Henry Martyn, Robert Morrison, Samuel Marsden, Christian Frederick Schwartz, David Livingston, Robert Murray M'Cheyne, Andrew Murray, Sheldon Jackson and Jim Elliot to name just a few people.[1]

He ministered mostly in the northeast United States to the Native Americans. Sadly, his ministry was cut short by his untimely death at the young age of twenty-nine. He wrestled with mental and physical illness his whole life. On Sunday, February 3, 1745, for example, he wrote about his depression:

> My soul remembered "the wormwood and the gall" . . . of Friday last; and I was greatly afraid . . . and made me long for the grave more, unspeakably more, than for hid treasures.[2]

As you read his journals, you will see over and over his battle with deep, dark depression. His struggle was so severe at times that he longed for death. He documented his longing for death about twenty-one times.[3]

What if Brainerd's journals were not just a documentation of his walk with God? What if they were also his counselor? What if journaling was a tool that God used to help him process the pain within? And what if that same tool, journaling, could also help us process our pain?

The Medicine of Journaling

In Bible college, a professor assigned journaling to my class as an assignment for spiritual growth. Little did I know what a blessing it would be. I have engaged in this spiritual practice ever since. I think of journaling as a practical way to follow the example of Moses. "At the LORD's command Moses recorded the stages in their journey. This is their journey by stages" (Numbers 33:2). Just as Moses recorded the physical journey of the Israelites, journaling is a way to record your spiritual journey.

In addition, journaling has helped me manage my mind and process my emotions. I call it "paper therapy." Anne Frank said, "Paper has more patience than people."[4] Time and time again, I have found this to be true; therefore, my journal is my counselor, my friend, and my clarifier!

I agree with Ronald Klug, who wrote:

> A journal or diary . . . is a daybook—a place to record daily happenings. But it is far more than that. A journal is also a tool for

self-discovery, an aid to concentration, a mirror for the soul, a place to generate and capture ideas, a safety valve for the emotions, a training ground for the writer, and a good friend and confidant.[5]

Out of all the mental health tools I share in this book, journaling is one of my favorites. I hope you will give it a try.

Barriers to Journaling

You might think that you're not a good writer, but journaling isn't about being a good writer. It's about ordering your mind and processing your thoughts. Journaling helps me bring order to my mind when it is in a state of chaos.

"I don't have time to journal," you say. Do you have time to worry and stew? Do you have time to ruminate? Do you have time to think scary thoughts? If you have time to worry, you have time to write. If you have time to ruminate, you have time to reflect. The time spent journaling will cut down on the time spent worrying.

You say, "I don't have good penmanship." Penmanship is not the point. Processing your thoughts is. Dawson Trotman, the founder of the Navigators, once quipped, "Thoughts disentangle themselves when they pass through the lips and the fingertips."[6]

My Favorite Journaling Tools

When you become aware that you are triggered, anxious, or angry, push the pause button and take out your journal.

ABCDE. Process what is going on in your heart with these five steps:

1. *Awareness*. The first step is self-awareness. "Examine yourselves" (2 Corinthians 13:5). Write down what happened and your emotional response to it. Express your emotions on paper. "I feel angry that they cut me off in traffic."

2. *Bear.* The second step is proactively accepting your feelings as a temporary psychological reality. Endure them with grace. "I choose to bear this anger and choose to lean into it with God's help."

3. *Call.* The third step is to ask God for His guidance. Pray, *Lord, help me see what is really going on.*

4. *Dissect.* The fourth step is to put on your investigator hat and ask, "Why do I feel this way? Why is this bothering me? What core fear is this situation tapping into?" After asking why questions to discern the causes of your triggered state, challenge yourself with questions like, What is the truth? What thoughts are leading to this feeling?

   The reason this step is so powerful is because it taps into what Martin Seligman calls "explanatory style." This is how you explain the happenings of your life. It is how you interpret what happens to you. Dr. Seligman found a connection between depression and explanatory style. "People who made certain kind of explanations . . . are prey to helplessness. Teaching them to change these explanations might prove an effective way to treat their depression."[7] In this step, you examine your explanations of events and ask yourself if those explanations are true.

5. *Engage.* After investigating the situation, ask the Lord how He wants you to respond. "If any of you lacks wisdom, you should ask God, who gives generously to all without finding fault, and it will be given to you" (James 1:5).

What is bothering me? In *The Coaching Habit,* Michael Bungay Stanier cites a study that found that "any time we have something on our mind, it's literally using up energy—even though it accounts for only about 2 percent of your body weight, your brain uses about 20 percent of your energy."[8] If something is weighing on your mind, it is wasting valuable energy. A helpful exercise to do is called "What is bothering me?"

First, at the top of a sheet of paper, write this question: What is bothering me? Make a list of what is bothering you. Next, one by one, go over the list, asking, Can I change this situation?

If not, hand it over to God. Surrender it to Him. Say something like, *Lord, I give You this problem.* If it is within your power to do something about the situation, pray, *Lord, what do You want me to do about it*? Write down what He tells you to do and obey His guidance.

The morning download. After waking up in the morning, my mind often races over all the things I must do that day. I need to call Jim today, work on my sermon, and walk the dogs. What if this happens? What if that happens?

A helpful journaling tool I've discovered is to write down all those thoughts on a piece of paper. I call this my "morning download." I don't evaluate what I am writing, I just unload all those thoughts on a piece of paper. Afterward, I feel much calmer and more centered. I will then pray a prayer, *Lord, I give You these worries and cares. Please give me Your peace.*

Scripture writing. This is writing down God's Word in your journal, copying it word for word. I have found that it helps me slow down and immerse myself in a text more fully. It helps me marinate my soul more fully in God's Word.

Slow Thinking—Fast Thinking

In *Thinking Fast and Slow*, Daniel Kahneman explains two thinking modes. The first mode is what he calls fast mode where we react quickly to the happenings of our lives. He says that since we live in such a fast-paced environment, we often live in this zone.

The second thinking mode is the slow mode. This is a deeper, more reflective mode of thinking. It is when we contemplate a problem or a strategy, mulling it over, and seeing it from different angles and viewpoints.

He has discovered that spending time in the slow mode dramatically affects how we react in the fast mode. Slow thinking is training for fast thinking. It is the practice before the game.[9]

There are volumes of neuroscience behind this phenomenon: Slow thinking taps into a whole different section of our brain. The synapses literally fire differently. We know that great leaders learn to train their default state through scheduled times of thinking slowly, deliberately, and intentionally.[10]

BEYOND THE BOOK

Takeaway: Practice paper therapy.

Verse to memorize: "Write this down" (Revelation 21:5).

Question to consider: What is keeping you from journaling?

Reflections: _____

_____

_____

_____

_____

Prayer: *Lord Jesus, sometimes my mind feels messy. It feels out of sorts. During those times, help me to bring order to my mind by downloading my cares and concerns on paper. As I do, please give me Your peace and perspective. Please give me the joy of journaling. By faith, I chose to practice paper therapy, knowing it's not the paper that brings healing but Your Spirit. Paper is a tool—You are the healer. Amen.*

Application: Pick one of these journaling exercises in this chapter and use it today:

- ABCDE
- What is bothering me?
- Morning download
- Scripture writing

CHAPTER FOURTEEN

The Test of the Truth

Then you will know the truth, and the truth will set you free.

John 8:32

"I am worn out from this struggle," she said with tears in her eyes. I could feel the anxiety in her soul as she shared her struggle with me. Her husband sat next to her, holding her hand.

"What is going on?" I asked in a curious tone.

"A few months ago, I felt something switch in my spirit," she said. "I went from being carefree to feeling locked in my mind. I am wrestling with paralyzing anxiety." She picked at her fingers and fidgeted in her chair as she said those words.

"I want my wife back," the husband said. You could hear the desperation in his voice. "We are here because we don't know what to do."

As I looked at these two faithful followers of Jesus, my spirit welled with compassion. I put on my listening hat and sought to understand more about the situation.

"I haven't left the house. I haven't driven my car since I have been in this fearful place." Next, she asked a question that I could see was weighing on her mind. "What is causing this? Is this because of Satan? Is my mental anguish coming from a satanic attack?"

If you wrestle with mental illness, or know someone who does, you have probably asked the same question—is Satan the cause of my mental illness?

Satan's Job Description

If Satan had a job description, here is how it might read: Your job is to steal, kill, and destroy God's children by the following methods:

- Tempt—Matthew 4:3; 1 Thessalonians 3:5
- Accuse—Revelation 12:10
- Oppose God's work—Matthew 16:23
- Bring suffering—Luke 13:16
- Fight against the church—Ephesians 6:11–12
- Deception—John 8:44

Satan Lies to Us

Of all his tactics, I think his most potent one is deception. He is called the father of lies.

> For you are the children of your father the devil, and you love to do the evil things he does. He was a murderer from the beginning. He has always hated the truth, because there is no truth in him. When he lies, it is consistent with his character; for he is a liar and the father of lies.
>
> John 8:44 NLT

When Satan lies, he is speaking his mother tongue. Is it possible that you are caught in a cobweb of his lies?

Recall when Jesus told Peter about His upcoming death and resurrection. How did Peter respond? "Peter took him aside and began to rebuke him. 'Never, Lord!' he said. 'This shall never happen to you'" (Matthew 16:22). Peter's view of the Messiah did not include suffering, so he challenges Jesus.

Jesus sees what is happening in the invisible realm. Satan is trying to use Peter to thwart His mission. He responds, "Get behind me, Satan! You are a stumbling block to me; you do not have in mind the concerns of God, but merely human concerns" (Matthew 16:23).

Is Jesus calling Peter Satan? One minute He calls Peter the Rock, and the next minute, He calls him Satan?

No.

Jesus is not calling Peter Satan. He is recognizing the source of Peter's thoughts. Satan had planted those thoughts in Peter's mind.

Are you aware that Satan can plant toxic thoughts in your mind? This is why it is so important to take your thoughts captive and then ask yourself if they are true.

The Truth Shall Set You Free

The Layman's Bible Dictionary defines truth as, "That which is reliable and consistent with God's revelation."[1] Since God's revelation is recorded in the Bible, we need to filter our thoughts and make sure they align with God's thoughts. As followers of Jesus, we believe something is true to the degree that it aligns with the Bible's teachings. "Sanctify them by the truth; your word is truth" (John 17:17).

Locating Lies and Replacing Them

Ponder when Satan tempted Jesus in the wilderness. How did He respond to Satan's lies? "It is written" (Matthew 4:4). Jesus countered Satan's lies with God's truth. A wise person follows His example. Here are three ways to replace Satan's lies with God's truth:[2]

Locating the lies. As I have shared in this book, our church was going through a very difficult season in 2002. During this season, a few people expressed their doubt about my leadership ability. I assumed the few were speaking for the majority. This caused me to doubt myself.

Going against my overseer's advice, I called for a vote of confidence from the church. I gave people the opportunity to vote on whether or not they trusted me as their leader. To my surprise, the vote came back at 97 percent vote of confidence.

Looking back, I was absolutely convinced the majority didn't trust me. My mind told me this over and over. It was wrong. I believe that Satan planted that deceptive seed of thought in my mind, and I watered it by thinking obsessively about it. It kept me up at night. The good news is that, when I learned of its presence in my mind, I was able to cast it out. Is it possible that the devil has deceived you and you are totally oblivious to it? I recommend that you pray, *Holy Spirit, please show me a lie I am believing. Bring it out of the darkness and into the light.*

Replace lies with the truth. Once I learned that most of the congregation trusted me as their leader, I affirmed that truth in my mind. I thought about that 97 percent number over and over. I affirmed that truth as I went through the day.

Another way to affirm the truth of your situation is to ask the Holy Spirit to give you a promise from God's Word that you can focus on. Contemplate this thought so often that it becomes uppermost in your mind. If you feel insecure, for example, deeply muse on God's truth, "'Not by might nor by power, but by my Spirit,' says the Lord" (Zechariah 4:6).

Argue against the lie. "Finally, brothers and sisters, whatever is true, whatever is noble, whatever is right, whatever is pure, whatever is lovely, whatever is admirable—if anything is excellent or praiseworthy—think about such things" (Philippians 4:8). Paul gives the Philippians church a menu of healthy thoughts. Becky Meyerson calls this TNR PLA:[3]

True?
Noble?
Right?

Pure?

Lovely?

Admirable?

Imagine if you filtered all your thoughts through those six questions! It is true, noble, right, etc. If it doesn't align, argue against it.

Mental Illness or Demon Possession

Earlier, I shared the story about the lady who was confused about the source of her mental woes.

"Is what I am going through mental illness or demonic oppression?" she asked. Satanic beings can have an impact on our lives. "Physical situations may well be caused, controlled, or instigated by spiritual beings," wrote Robert Clinton.[4] They can also have an impact on our mental health.

> Mental disorders are complex states that result from an interaction of biology and environment. If we accept the argument that demons are presently active, then it is likely they are involved in some cases of mental illness. Demons are involved at many levels of our existence, and it certainly isn't necessary for demonic powers to purposefully cause a given mental illness in a person for us to be able to say that they were involved in the disorder.[5]

If you believe the root cause of your illness is satanic, use these three spiritual weapons:

- The name of Jesus (see Philippians 2:10)
- The blood of Jesus (see Revelation 12:11)
- The Word of God (see Ephesians 6:17)

Declare in faith, "Greater is he that is in you, than he that is in the world" (1 John 4:4 KJV). Satan is no match for your Savior! Be aware of Satan's wiles but keep your eyes on Jesus.

If you are unsure about the cause of your mental illness, consider this. The late Dr. Archibald Hart, author and former board member of the American Association of Christian Counselors, shares the following wisdom:

> Consider obvious causes first . . . for instance, if there is a history of mental illness in the family and the person you are counseling is experiencing bizarre behavior or emotions, the most likely cause is the family pattern of illness. Genetic factors strongly influence severe mental disorders. Unless you are trained in psychopathology, however, the most responsible action you can take is to refer the troubled person to a psychologist or psychiatrist for diagnosis.[6]

BEYOND THE BOOK

Takeaway: Don't automatically believe the thoughts that come into your mind. Rather, filter them through this question: Is it true?

Verse to memorize: "We demolish arguments and every pretension that sets itself up against the knowledge of God, and we take captive every thought to make it obedient to Christ" (2 Corinthians 10:5).

Questions to consider: What lies am I believing? And what is the truth of God's Word?

Reflections: _____

_____

_____

_____

Prayer: *Lord Jesus, I acknowledge that I have an enemy, and he is the father of lies. Please help me see the cobweb of lies I may be stuck in.*

Help me to replace his lies with Your truth. I affirm the truth of Your Word that says, "Then you will know the truth, and the truth will set you free." By faith, I choose to use the Word of God, the blood of Jesus, and the name of Jesus as my weapons against him. Amen.

Application: Ask the Holy Spirit to uncover a lie you are believing. After He has brought one to the surface, use the three steps from this chapter to replace the lie with God's truth.

Locate the lie

Replace the lie with God's truth

Argue against the lie

What was most useful to you about this exercise?

CHAPTER FIFTEEN

The Cause for Contentment

We have different gifts, according to the grace given to each of us.

Romans 12:6

"Lord, help me to be more like Billy Graham," Clarence prayed. He spent time at the altar asking God to make him more like his role model. As he did, he sensed God would not answer that prayer. Then the Spirit spoke to him, saying, "I won't do that. I've already got a Billy Graham. I want you to be you."

That was a life-altering moment in young Clarence's life. He told me that story over eggs, coffee, and fellowship at a local restaurant.

"Since that moment, I have been on a journey to be me."

Clarence's words challenged me to quit trying to be a second-class version of someone else and to start becoming a first-class version of who God made me to be. I vowed to quit striving to be someone other than who God made me to be. I started to appreciate my unique divine design.

Are you striving to be someone other than who God made you to be? Are you doubting God's sovereign choice to make you precisely how you are?

The Three Boxes

Imagine a series of boxes containing different gifts. The blue box contains musical ability, people skills, and leadership qualities. The green box contains writing, athletics, and mathematics. The red box contains management, public speaking, and working with your hands.

Imagine the blue box thinking, *I wish I had the talents that the green box has.* The blue box doesn't know that there is a good chance the green box may be thinking the same thoughts. Instead of focusing on what is in their box, *both boxes* are focused on what is *not* in their box. Are you making the same mistake?

The wiser path is to open your box with curiosity and awe, explore what God has sovereignly put in it, and then develop and deploy those gifts in the service of His kingdom. Paul writes to his protégé, Timothy, these words: "For this reason I remind you to fan into flame the gift of God, which is in you through the laying on of my hands" (2 Timothy 1:6). He is encouraging and exhorting him to use the gifts he has. Are you fanning into a flame the gifts God has given you? Or are you jealously focused on the gifts He has given others?

After researching leadership for over thirty years, Don Clifton says that appreciating the gifts in your box is his most important discovery:

> A leader needs to know his strengths as a carpenter knows his tools, or as a physician knows the instruments at her disposal. What great leaders have in common is that each truly knows his or her strengths—and can call on the right strength at the right time. This explains why there is no definitive list of characteristics that describes all leaders.[1]

Weakness Obsession

For much of my life, I had a "weakness obsession." I would obsess over what I wasn't good at and shame myself for not having certain gifts. *I should be more outgoing, more expressive, and more decisive.*

Do you have a weakness obsession? If so, what if you were to join me in asking God to give us a strengths focus? Imagine if we were aware of our weaknesses and developed ways to mitigate them, but our predominant focus became strengthening our strengths. This is important because you will be average—at best—in your weaknesses. But you can be world-class in your strengths. Do you want to be average or world-class?

When I Am Weak, He Is Strong

There is no way God could use me with my mental health struggles, you think. Wrong! One of the most comforting truths I have learned in my walk with God is that when I am weak, He is strong (see 2 Corinthians 12:10). My weakness is a platform for His glory! Henry Blackaby writes:

> God delights in using ordinary people to accomplish His divine purposes. Paul said God deliberately seeks out the weak and the despised things because it is from them that He receives the greatest glory. . . . When God does exceptional things through unexceptional people, then others recognize that only God could have done it. If you feel weak, limited, ordinary, take heart! You are the best material through which God can work![2]

Do you feel weak, limited, and ordinary? What if that makes you the ideal candidate for God to use for His glory?

David is a great example of a broken leader God used powerfully. "There in those caves, drowned in the sorrow of his song and in the song of his sorrow, David became the greatest hymn writer and the greatest comforter of broken hearts this world shall ever know."[3] Perhaps God wants to use your brokenness to bless others like David.

The Cause for Contentment

Perhaps you are wondering what being strengths-focused has to do with mental health. A lot.

In his book *Natural Church Development*, Christian Schwarz studied one thousand churches on five continents, looking for characteristics of healthy churches. He found eight. One of the characteristics was "gift-oriented ministry." In other words, in healthy churches, people were encouraged to discover the gifts God had placed in their box and use them to serve God by serving others. During that process, he made an exciting discovery:

> An interesting corollary result of our research was the discovery that probably no factor influences the contentedness of Christians more than whether they are utilizing their gifts or not. Our data demonstrated a highly significant relationship between "gift orientation" . . . and "joy in living."[4]

According to Schwarz, the number one factor in contented, joyful Christians is whether or not they know what gifts and talents God has placed in their boxes and if they are using them to serve and help others.

Starting today, I want you to begin the exciting journey of learning what God has placed in your box. To do that, you need to discover your natural gifts and spiritual gifts.

Natural gifts. When you were born, God placed natural abilities in your box. Psychologist Howard Gardner, in *Frames of Mind*,[5] lists seven natural abilities:

1. Logical-mathematical: Are you gifted with numbers? Are you an extremely logical thinker?

2. Verbal-linguistic: Are you gifted with words? Do you enjoy writing? Do you enjoy communicating?

3. Spatial-mechanical: Are you gifted at designing things? Are you an engineer at heart?

4. Musical: Are you gifted in music? When you sing and play an instrument, do you feel alive?

5. Bodily-kinesthetic: Are you gifted athletically? Can you do things with your body naturally that others can't?

6. Interpersonal-social: Are you naturally talented with people? Do you have a way with people?

7. Intrapersonal (self-knowledge): Are you aware of your inner world? Do you like to spend time in your inner space?

Spiritual gifts. If you are a genuine follower of Jesus, God has given you spiritual gifts. In the original language, spiritual gift means "grace gift." Spiritual gifts are not something you earn. They are given to you by grace. God puts these gifts in your box so that you can help build His church. They are meant for spiritual purposes. Henry Blackaby says that a spiritual gift is "a supernatural empowering to accomplish the assignment God gives you."[6]

Since we have different assignments, we have different gifts. Paul teaches:

We have different gifts, according to the grace given to each of us. If your gift is prophesying, then prophesy in accordance with your faith; if it is serving, then serve; if it is teaching, then teach; if it is to encourage, then give encouragement; if it is giving, then give generously; if it is to lead, do it diligently; if it is to show mercy, do it cheerfully.

Romans 12:6–8

God loves variety. He has a whole range of different gifts He distributes to His children:

Wisdom
Knowledge
Faith
Healing
Miracles
Prophecy
Discernment
Speaking in tongues
Interpretation of tongues

How Do You Discover Your Spiritual Gifts?

Experiment. A professor in college told me that we should put our hands on the plow and see if God blesses it. Experiment with different ministries. As you do, ask two questions: Is this rewarding? Is God blessing it?

Educate. The Bible contains many passages on spiritual gifts. Carve out time to study them and learn what God says. Read the following passages:

Romans 12:6–8
1 Corinthians 12:4–11
Ephesians 4:11–13

Examine. Take a spiritual gift inventory.

In 1981, a movie called *Chariots of Fire* told the story of a devout follower of Jesus named Eric Liddell who ran in the 1924 Olympics. His faith and passion for running collided when his 100-meter race was held on Sunday. He chose not to run that race because it would violate his practice of observing the Sabbath. He later ran in the 400-meter race and set a world record.

At one point in the film, Liddell says these thought-provoking words, "I believe that God made me for a purpose, but He also made me fast. And when I run, I feel His pleasure."[7]

Are you experiencing God's pleasure in your life because you are using the gifts He has placed in your box?

BEYOND THE BOOK

Takeaway: What gifts has God put in your box? How can you use them to serve others?

Verse to memorize: "We have different gifts, according to the grace given to each of us" (Romans 12:6).

Questions to consider: What gifts has God placed in your box? What are your natural abilities? What are your spiritual gifts? If you don't know, what will be your action plan to find out?

Reflections: ....

....

....

....

....

....

Prayer: *Lord Jesus, forgive me for the times I have tried to be someone I am not instead of who You created me to be. Please help me quit comparing myself to others and envying the gifts You've sovereignly placed in their box, and instead, help me to discover, develop, and deploy the gifts You've put in my box. Today, I choose to begin the journey of being me. Amen.*

Application: Do a joy experiment. After you have discovered your gifts, proactively spend time using them and note how you feel. Record your experience in a journal to see if using your gifts leads to greater contentment.

PART THREE

The Physical Key

Love the Lord your God . . . with all your strength.

Mark 12:30

CHAPTER SIXTEEN

The Effects of Exercise

After six days Jesus took with him Peter, James and John the brother of James, and led them up a high mountain by themselves.

Matthew 17:1

"How long have you been feeling this way?" a nurse asked. She took my vitals, recorded the results, and exited the room.

While waiting for the doctor, I observed the sterile hospital room with white walls and a patient bed. I pondered my extreme fatigue. I didn't have the energy to make it through the day unless I took a long nap and drank several cups of coffee.

Knock, knock. In came the doctor.

"Hello, Pastor Larson," he greeted. He was wearing a white coat and had a stethoscope wrapped around his neck. He asked me a series of questions. As he did, I revealed that I had stopped exercising.

"Why did you stop exercising?" he questioned.

"A doctor recommended it. I saw him a few weeks ago and told him that I was wrestling with a bad cold. He told me to stop exercising."

"How long ago did you stop exercising?"

"Two weeks ago."

"How long have you been feeling more fatigued and depressed?"

"About two weeks." As he said those words, a lightbulb went on in my mind.

"Do you see the connection?" he asked. "The reason you are feeling so tired is because you quit exercising. You need to start again right away."

I left that appointment with a sense of hope. *If I start exercising, I will feel more energetic*, I thought.

It worked!

I began exercising again that day, and within no time, I started feeling more energetic and less depressed. I learned a valuable lesson: Motion affects emotions. Moving your body stimulates feel-good chemicals in your brain, while being sedentary makes you miss out on that natural "high."

Bodily Training Is of Some Value

"Rather train yourself for godliness; *for while bodily training is of some value,* godliness is of value in every way, as it holds promise for the present life and also for the life to come" (1 Timothy 4:7–8 ESV, emphasis added).

In this text, Paul tells Timothy to train to become godly because godliness has value in this life and eternity. He also mentions that physical training, or exercise, has value. He prioritizes spiritual fitness over physical fitness. He does say, however, that exercise has value. Do you see exercise as a worthwhile, valuable activity?

In my early twenties, I neglected exercise because I saw it as unspiritual. I thought I could be doing more spiritual things, like prayer, Bible study, or witnessing. Ironically, I have learned that exercising gives me more energy to do spiritual things—pray, read my Bible, and reflect Christ's love to this world.

The Effects of Exercise

Here are five benefits of practicing daily exercise:

It sharpens our brain. Did you know that physical exercise builds and strengthens your brain? In the book *Spark*, the authors write:

The brain responds like muscles do, growing with use, withering with inactivity. The neurons in the brain connect to one another through "leaves" on treelike branches, and exercise causes those branches to grow and bloom with new buds, thus enhancing brain function at a fundamental level.[1]

If you want a stronger, healthier brain, exercise your body. An example of this can be found at a school in Chicago—Naperville Central High School. The school incorporated a morning exercise program for students called Zero Hour. They found that the students who participated in the hour of exercise before school saw "a 17 percent improvement in reading and comprehension, compared with a 10.7 percent improvement among the other literary students who opted to sleep in and take standard phys ed."[2]

It increases our energy. "Give, and it will be given to you. A good measure, pressed down, shaken together and running over, will be poured into your lap. For with the measure you use, it will be measured to you" (Luke 6:38).

This verse teaches a counterintuitive truth: It is in giving that we receive. I've learned this is true of exercise. The more energy I give to moving my body, the more energy and vitality I experience. Stephen Covey says:

> Most of us think we don't have enough time to exercise. What a distorted paradigm! We don't have time not to. We're talking about three to six hours a week—or a minimum of thirty minutes a day, every other day. That hardly seems an inordinate amount of time considering the tremendous benefits in terms of the impact on the other 162–165 hours of the week."[3]

It shows gratitude to God. God has given us the gift of our physical nature, and when we take care of it, we show gratitude to the giver of the gift. It is an act of worship. Imagine praying a prayer like this as you exercise: *God thank you for the ability to walk, run, and squat. Thank you for this body you have given me. I want to take care of it so I can serve you longer.*

It can help you serve God better and longer. The better you care for your vehicle, the longer it will last. Getting regular oil changes, making sure the tires are filled, and having regular tune-ups prolong the life of the vehicle. In general, the same is true of our body. The better we take care of ourselves, the longer we will live. "You've got only one body; you need to take care of it," my 93-year-old dad has said to me my whole life. He is a good example of being a good steward of his health. He has always been active, a moderate eater, and avoids harmful substances like tobacco and alcohol.

It helps cope with depression and anxiety. In my earlier years, I exercised because I wanted to look good physically. Now I exercise because I want to feel good mentally. When I exercise, feel-good chemicals in my brain are stimulated. Often as I walk to my exercise room to ride the bike or lift weights, I tell myself, "I need a mental boost."

Jerry, a mentor of mine, said that one of his daily mantras is, "Just get moving." Whether he gets up to dust the living room, go for a walk, or play pickleball, he reminds himself to avoid being stationary.

It is so important to develop the mindset of moving because we live in a very sedentary culture. I have a friend who jokingly said, "My favorite form of exercise is power sitting." We sit too much and exercise too little.

I pray this chapter will inspire you to "become a cardiovascular Christian."[4] I pray that you will resist the modern culture's encouragement of inactivity and develop the daily habit of exercise.

Walking is one of the simplest and most powerful ways to exercise.

> Walking connects the right and left hemispheres of your brain, helping your brain get "unstuck." It releases endorphins and fires up your neurotransmitters, providing greater clarity of thought. . . . Walking regularly improves memory, fights rigidity in your brain, and helps long-term brain function and health in myriad ways.[5]

Here are some other tips on how to make exercise a regular part of your life:

- Talk to your doctor before you begin an exercise program. Get his or her input.
- Find an accountability partner. This should be someone who will exercise with you and encourage you in the process.
- Balance aerobic exercise with weightlifting.
- Discover your rhythm. Some people prefer exercising in the morning and others at night.
- Find something you enjoy.
- Take small steps. "I am going to walk for five minutes today," tell yourself. And then walk ten the next day.
- Exercise with God. Talk to Him as you walk through the woods. Turn your walks into worship. Sing when you're walking up the stairs.

Exercise—What Would Jesus Do?

Did Jesus exercise? According to Roger Reynolds in his "Just as I Am" wellness seminar, the answer is a resounding yes! Deborah Newman shares what she learned from his seminar:

> He measured the miles between cities that Jesus walked in His three years of open ministry and calculated that Jesus was in peak aerobic fitness. He also took into consideration that Jesus had been a carpenter and lumberjack, occupations that would have given him high levels of muscular endurance, strength, and flexibility.[6]

BEYOND THE BOOK

Takeaway: Exercising your body energizes your mind.

Verse to memorize: "Train yourself for godliness; for while bodily training is of some value, godliness is of value in every way, as it holds promise for the present life and also for the life to come" (1 Timothy 4:7–8 NIV).

Questions to consider: What are your most significant barriers to daily exercise, and how can you overcome them in the Lord?

Reflections: _____

_____

_____

_____

_____

_____

Prayer: *Lord, I wrestle with inactivity. Please inspire me to become more active. Please help me to appreciate the gift of movement, knowing that being able to move, walk, and exercise is an amazing privilege. By faith, I choose to stand more and sit less, get off the couch and onto the court, turn off the television and get on the treadmill for Your glory. Amen.*

Application: Make a list of all the possible ways you could get exercise. Experiment with each one and record how well you enjoyed it. Look for 3–4 modes of exercise that you really enjoy doing.

Exercise	Enjoyment Scale (1 = Miserable, 5 = enjoyable)
Pickleball	4
Hiking	2
Rucking	5
Bike riding	2
Basketball	1

CHAPTER SEVENTEEN

The Nature of Nutrition

Jesus came, took the bread and gave it to them, and did the same with the fish.

John 21:13

"How are you doing?" I asked. I was meeting a mentor of mine at a restaurant to catch up. As we were talking, the waitress asked for our order.

"I will have a hamburger and fries," I said, closing my menu and giving it to her. I glanced out the window and saw vehicles driving by on the highway as the incoming sunshine warmed my face.

"I will have a salad," said my mentor.

A salad, I thought. I had eaten with him many times before, and the last thing he would have ordered would have been a salad. I doubt it had ever crossed his mind.

"Are you on a diet?" I asked. He paused for a moment and put his drink down.

"Yes. For many years, I neglected my health and ate whatever I wanted." I could hear regret oozing out of his heart. "That is catching up with me. I have decided to make better health choices."

I felt guilty for having ordered a greasy hamburger and fries.

As he put the green salad in his mouth, he said, "Every bite is an act of worship."

Eating is an act of worship! I had never made that connection before. Have you? Do you see your nutritional choices as an act of worship? "So whether you eat or drink or whatever you do, do it all for the glory of God" (1 Corinthians 10:31).

What if we began to eat for God's glory? Imagine if we saw every bite as an act of worship.

Every Meal Is Medicine

Growing up near Rochester, Minnesota, I received health care from the Mayo Clinic. It is one of the most prestigious hospitals in the world, and people fly in from all over the world to receive medical help. God has used the Mayo Clinic to save both my dad's life and my younger brother's life.

Just as the Mayo Clinic helps people in the medical realm, what if there is a branch of medicine that we overlook every day? Hippocrates, an ancient Greek physician and philosopher, said, "Let food be thy medicine and medicine be thy food."[1] Imagine if we saw food as medicine. Imagine if we made food choices based on nutritional value, asking, "Will this meal move me toward a healthier self?" Here are seven steps to making wise food choices:

Food affects mood. Did you know there is a connection between the food that you eat and your mood? The food you eat influences the feelings you feel. Think about Elijah's depression. After experiencing a mountaintop victory on Mount Carmel, he sinks into a deep depression and prays to die. Interestingly, the ministering angels tell him to get proper nutrition. "Then he lay down under the bush and fell asleep. All at once an angel touched him and said, '*Get up and eat*'" (1 Kings 19:5, emphasis added).

The angel prescribed nutrition for Elijah's mental anguish. He knew that proper nutrition was a part of his healing journey.

Have you made the connection between the foods you eat and the moods you feel? Do you see your nutritional choices as a pathway to better mental health? An article in *Psychology Today* drives home the connection between food and mood. After citing reasons why food affects mood, the author summarizes the article by saying:

> The foods that we eat do affect our moods, feelings, and cognitive function. A diet focused on fruits and vegetables, lean proteins and whole grains can help to boost mental health. And specific supplements and diets are proven to help with certain mental health conditions.[2]

Eat God's food, not man's food. "What kind of food should I eat?" you ask. In *The Daniel Plan,* Rick Warren writes, "Our philosophy is that if it was grown on a plant, eat it. If it was made in a plant, leave it on the shelf."[3] Eat God-formed food, not human-processed food. Eat food that is "whole, fresh, and unprocessed."[4]

Look to Christ for comfort, not food. What is the purpose of food? Have you ever pondered that question? Why did God create food?

Some people use food as an emotional comforter. They call it comfort food. They open the fridge when they are stressed and anxious. They reach for ice cream when feeling down, desiring the temporary high it brings.

Regretfully, I have fallen into this pattern many times in my life. I have reached for a bag of chips to make me happy instead of God. Is food your comforter?

Other people see food as fuel. Its purpose is to meet their nutritional needs, not their emotional and spiritual ones. What about you? What is your relationship with food? Do a little experiment with me. Before eating, ask, "Why am I eating this? For fuel? Or comfort?" You may be surprised how often you expect food to do what only God can do. Only God can satisfy the longing of your heart. Perhaps that is why Jesus said, "I am the bread of life. Whoever comes to me will never go hungry, and whoever believes in me will never be thirsty" (John 6:35).

Imagine if we looked to bread to meet our nutritional needs and looked to the bread of life—Jesus—to meet our spiritual needs!

Imagine if we honestly searched our hearts and asked this uncomfortable question, "Have I made food my idol? Have I given it Godlike power in my life?" In his book, *The Maker's Diet,* Jordan Rubin writes, "In our era, we have allowed food to become our idol. Too many people admittedly 'live to eat.'"[5]

The Bible does not teach, "Taste and see that the Snickers Bar and Pepsi are good." Instead, it teaches, "Taste and see that the LORD is good" (Psalm 34:8).

If food has become your idol, pray,

God, please forgive me for making food my idol. As of today, I look to food to meet my nutritional needs and to You to meet my spiritual needs. By faith, I choose to look to You for comfort, not food. Please satisfy the deep longings of my heart. In Jesus' name, Amen.

Develop self-control. "But the fruit of the Spirit is love, joy, peace, forbearance, kindness, goodness, faithfulness, gentleness and self-control" (Galatians 5:22–23).

Self-control is a fruit of the Spirit. As you abide in Jesus, He will give you the power to control yourself. This is crucial when it comes to food because we live in a world that scripts us to practice gluttony and overindulge our appetites. Do you need to pray, *Lord, help me to control my dietary urges and not allow them to control me?*

- Proverbs 25:16: "If you find honey, eat just enough—too much of it, and you will vomit."
- Proverbs 23:20–21: "Do not join those who drink too much wine or gorge themselves on meat, for drunkards and gluttons become poor, and drowsiness clothes them in rags."
- Philippians 3:19: "Their destiny is destruction, their god is their stomach, and their glory is in their shame. Their mind is set on earthly things."

Eat with an eye for the future. Many years ago, I came across a formula that helps me consider the future consequences of my present choices. It's called 10-10-10. It asks, "What will be the consequence of this choice in 10 minutes, 10 months, and 10 years?"

Imagine if we applied that formula to the food we eat. What will be the consequence of a habitual diet of junk food in . . .

- 10 minutes: I will have a sugar high followed by a crash.
- 10 months: I may be overweight or obese.
- 10 years: I may develop diabetes.

Ask God to help you eat with an eye for the future. Here's why this is important:

> Research now shows that the majority of Americans today are malnourished. But it's not because we're underfed. If anything, we're probably overfed. Our problem is hidden starvation; the foods we eat every day are actually killing us.[6]

Stop at 80 percent. Dan Buettner shares the results of a study he did on longevity. He studied the "Blue Zones," where people had the highest life expectancies. Looking for their secrets to longevity, he found an interesting habit from the people of Okinawa, Japan. One of the secrets he discovered can be summarized in the phrase *Hara hachi bu*. It means to "stop eating when you're 80% full."[7] They stop eating when they are 80 percent full. Instead of gorging themselves, they control themselves. Imagine asking the Lord to give you the self-control to stop eating when you are 80 percent full.

Eat like Jesus. "What would Jesus do?" is a question Christians often ask themselves. WWJD is the abbreviated form of that question. It's a great question. What if we also asked, "What would Jesus eat?"

Have you ever pondered Jesus' diet? He ate a Mediterranean diet of nuts, fruits, and grains. He often fed people broiled fish and whole-grain bread. After examining Jesus' diet, one author concluded, "Jesus ate in a healthful manner."[8]

Imagine putting a bracelet around your wrist that said WWJE— What Would Jesus Eat?

BEYOND THE BOOK

Takeaway: Every bite is an act of worship.

Verse to memorize: "Then he lay down under the bush and fell asleep. All at once an angel touched him and said, 'Get up and eat'" (1 Kings 19:5).

Questions to consider: Have you turned food into an idol? Do you see food as fuel or comfort?

Reflections:

_____

_____

_____

_____

_____

Prayer: *Lord, forgive me for turning to food for comfort when I should be turning to You. Help me put food in its proper place, seeing it as fuel for the body rather than comfort for my soul. Help me choose my food based on its nutritional value rather than my emotional state. Help me to eat more food from the garden and less from the factory. By faith, I chose to make healthy food choices, remembering that every bite is an act of worship.*

Application: Keep a food log. Write down what you eat and why you eat it. Do this for a few days and see what you learn.

CHAPTER EIGHTEEN

The Habit of Hydration

When a Samaritan woman came to draw water, Jesus said to her, "Will you give me a drink?"

John 4:7

What happened? I was lying on my back in a dazed state. I could feel the dry grass tickling my neck. *Where am I?* was my next thought.

"Are you okay?" a coworker asked me with genuine concern.

"I am okay," I responded. "What happened?"

"You passed out."

This event happened in my early teens when I worked for a beekeeper. I enjoyed many aspects of the job—being out in nature, the camaraderie of my coworkers, and strengthening my muscles through hard work. There was, however, one thing I did not like: extracting, or taking parts of bees' homes away, so that harvesting them for honey was possible.

On the hot summer day that I passed out, I was extracting. With adrenaline pumping through my body, I wore a snowmobile-like suit for protection. Being so engrossed in my work, I made a serious health mistake. I didn't drink enough water.

After I came to, my coworker led me into a white farmhouse where I lay in front of a fan and drank lots of water. My mouth felt as dry as the Sahara Desert, and I was dizzy and highly fatigued.

That day, I learned valuable lessons: stay hydrated, drink water regularly, and be on guard against dehydration.

Do you value getting enough water? Do you understand water's importance to your overall health and well-being? Dr. Don Colbert, an American physician, author, and speaker, wrote, "Water is the single most important nutrient for our bodies. It is involved in every function of our bodies. You can live five to seven weeks without food, but the average adult can last no more than five days without water."[1]

Many people do not value water as they should, and as a result, they are dehydrated. Being dehydrated is dangerous. One of the simplest ways to improve your overall health is to drink enough water daily. It is a small step that can have massive rewards. That is why I am encouraging you to develop the habit of hydration.

Hydration and Mental Wellness

Being properly hydrated is essential for your mental wellness.

Studies show that you only need to be 1% dehydrated to experience a 5% decrease in cognitive function. A 2% decrease in brain hydration can result in short term memory loss and have trouble with math computations. Prolonged dehydration causes brain cells to shrink in size and mass, a condition common in many elderly who have been dehydrated for years.[2]

In addition, proper hydration leads to higher levels of happiness.

Not drinking enough water can negatively affect your mood. Without water, the brain can't get enough of the amino acid tryptophan needed to create serotonin, also known as the "feel good" chemical. That's a big problem because serotonin is the neurotransmitter that regulates mood. Increasing your water intake will promote happiness, allowing your brain to continue making serotonin.[3]

If you want a healthier, happier brain, prioritize staying properly hydrated.

Symptoms of Dehydration

Since hydration is healthy and dehydration is dangerous, it is essential to recognize the signs of dehydration. Here are five signs of dehydration:

- Depression
- Afternoon fatigue
- Sleep issues
- Inability to focus
- Lack of mental clarity, sometimes referred to as "brain fog"[4]

Can you relate to any of these symptoms? If so, you may be dehydrated.

The Living Water

In the gospel of John, Jesus encounters a spiritually thirsty woman who tries to satisfy her inner thirst by forming relationships with men. She has been married five times, and the guy she is presently with is not her husband.

Jesus explains to her that having a relationship with Him is like drinking living water. "Everyone who drinks this water will be thirsty again, but whoever drinks the water I give them will never thirst. Indeed, the water I give them will become in them a spring of water welling up to eternal life" (John 4:13–14).

Isn't it interesting that Jesus compares Himself to water? Might that give us a hint of how important water is to our overall health?

Moreover, did you know that water is mentioned 722 times in the Bible? More than faith, hope, or worship.[5] If water is mentioned so often in the Bible, perhaps God is trying to communicate to us how important it is. Have you made the connection between staying hydrated and being healthy? Do you recognize the importance of water to your daily health?

How Much Water Should We Aim For?

How much water should we drink? What target should we aim for? "The National Academy of Medicine recommends that men consume 125 ounces (3,700 mL) and women about 90 ounces (2,700 mL) of fluid per day, including the fluid from water, other drinks, and foods."[6]

How to Develop the Habit of Hydration

"Sow a thought and you reap an action; sow an act and you reap a habit; sow a habit and you reap a character; sow a character and you reap a destiny." Those words are widely attributed Ralph Waldo Emerson, the American essayist, philosopher, and poet.

How do we develop the habit of hydration? Here are a few ideas:

Use cue cards. In the beginning of a new habit, it is important for you to put up reminders as prompts of the new habit. This is important because we know how easy it is for something to be out of sight, out of mind. One way to do this is to put cue cards in your environment that have the word *water* on them. You could, for example, write the word water on a 3x5 card and put it on your refrigerator or bathroom mirror.

Put a reminder on your phone. Program your phone to remind you to drink water every few hours. This way, you won't have to stress about remembering to drink enough water; your phone will do it for you.

Monitor the color of your urine. If your urine is dark, you need to drink more water. Aim to have pale yellow urine.

Carry a reusable water bottle with you throughout the day. Wherever you go, bring a reusable water bottle. Discipline yourself to take sips of it all day long. Don't wait until you are thirsty to drink. Aim to be a like a good waiter. They don't wait until your water glass is empty to refill it—they refill it before it is empty. Similarly, don't wait till you are thirsty to drink. Often, that is a sign that you are dehydrated. Drink proactively, not reactively.

Drink two glasses of water when you wake up. Upon waking up in the morning, discipline yourself to drink two glasses of water. Think about it. It has probably been six to eight hours since you last drank anything. You have some catching up to do. While your coffee is brewing, chug two glasses of water.

Flavor your water. Perhaps you don't enjoy the taste of water or get bored with its blandness. Try adding some healthy flavors to it, like lemon, cucumber, mint, or berries.

Eat foods that are saturated with water. Watermelon, oranges, strawberries, cucumbers, celery, and lettuce are examples of foods that are high in water saturation. Purposefully eat more of them to supplement your drinking.

Drink a glass of water before each meal. Before you eat, hydrate. One of the benefits of this practice is that it will help curb your appetite. Drinking water before you eat will give your stomach a sense of fullness, which will help you eat moderately. In addition, sometimes those hunger pangs are really thirst pangs. You reach for food when what you really need is water.

Blue Mind Theory

"Let's get going," my parents said. We jumped in the car and made the two-hour drive to Okoboji, Iowa.

"Are we there yet?" one of us kids would ask, anticipating the clear, blue lakes and sandy shorelines. As we entered Okoboji, we often saw a long line of trucks with their boats behind them. It was like seeing a parade of yachts, sailboats, and fishing boats. Laughter from people water-skiing could be heard for miles.

During my sabbatical in 2002, I spent a lot of time by the lakes. God used those lakes to heal my soul. I sat by the lake and talked to God for hours, all the while hearing the raspy, honking sound of a pelican flying over me and feeling the warm sand go through my toes. As a result, I find the sight of water extremely healing.

I am not alone.

Marine biologist Wallace Nichols developed the Blue Mind Theory,[7] which suggests that being near water or doing water-related activities can have a positive effect on your mental well-being.

The moral is clear: Don't just drink water; try to be around it as much as possible. It is good for your mental health.

Will you ask Jesus to help you develop the habit of hydration?

BEYOND THE BOOK

Takeaway: Develop the habit of hydration! A hydrated brain is a happier brain.

Verse to memorize: "When a Samaritan woman came to draw water, Jesus said to her, 'Will you give me a drink?'" (John 4:7).

Question to consider: How can I practice Blue Mind Theory and be around water more?

Reflections:

Prayer: *Lord, thank You for the gift of water. Please give me the discipline to drink frequently. As I drink water today, remind me that You are the living water for my soul. Also, thank You for the beauty of oceans, lakes, and streams. Fill my soul as I spend time around them. Amen.*

Application: Write down three ideas on how you can drink more water.

CHAPTER NINETEEN

The Duty of Delight

A cheerful heart is good medicine, but a crushed spirit dries up the bones.

Proverbs 17:22

During the uncertainty of the COVID-19 pandemic, I spiraled into a pit of despair and despondency. I was worried about the virus and its impact. *How deadly is it? How long will we be in lockdown? What will be its future implications?*

I set an appointment to see a counselor to stop the downward trajectory. After checking in, I sat in the waiting room. I could feel the anxiety in the air. People were fidgeting with their masks, not being used to them yet.

"What can I help you with?" the counselor asked. I shared with her the mental anguish I was feeling. She asked me a series of questions. One of them really caught me off guard.

"What do you do for fun?" she asked. I froze.

Fun? I thought. *What does that have to do with mental health? Besides, I don't have time for that.*

"I am not sure," I responded.

At that time in my life, I did not value recreation. I thought it was unspiritual and lazy. So I switched topics.

"I have been busy with ministry. However, the good news is that I have gotten a lot done." Then I listed some of my accomplishments.

"I know you are ambitious," she said before she paused. I could tell she was trying to choose her words carefully. "I want to encourage you to broaden your scope of ambition. What if you were to become ambitious about having fun?"

Ambitious about fun? That sounded like an oxymoron. Thoughts like that had never entered my mind.

As a recovering workaholic, I don't wake up in the morning and automatically think about having fun. *What do I need to do?* is where my mind tends to go. I tend to focus on improving the world, not enjoying it.

Thankfully, my wife is a great "fun mentor." She loves to have fun and is very adventurous. We often joke that her job is to make sure that we have fun; my job is to make sure we can pay the bills. Here are six ways to have more fun in life.

Develop a sense of humor. In *The Humor of Christ*, author and theologian Elton Trueblood points to an aspect of Jesus' personality that is easy to overlook: humor.[1] This is because the humor of our day and age differs significantly from the humor in His day and age. In our culture, humor is about telling jokes. Jewish humor, on the other hand, "often employed witty hyperbole—clever, startling, over-the-top statements—to get a laugh."[2]

An example of this is when Jesus said, "Do not throw your pearls to pigs" (Matthew 7:6). As we read that verse, we might think, *Why would anyone do that? That's ridiculous.* That's the point. The original hearers would have bellied over in laughter.

Trueblood notes:

There are numerous passages . . . which are practically incomprehensible when regarded as sober prose, but which are luminous once we become liberated from the gratuitous assumption that Christ never joked. . . . Once we realize that Christ was not always engaged in pious talk, we have made an enormous step on the road to understanding.[3]

Does your view of Jesus include His fun and humorous side? For many years, mine didn't. But make no mistake—He was.

Let children mentor you. "And he said: 'Truly I tell you, unless you change and become like little children, you will never enter the kingdom of heaven'" (Matthew 18:3). Jesus pointed to children as an example of childlike faith. Just as children trust their earthly fathers to care for them, we must trust our heavenly Father. What if children can teach us more than just childlike faith? What if they can also teach us about childlike fun? What if adults looked to children to learn how to have fun? Did you know that the average child laughs four hundred times a day, while the average adult laughs fifteen times?[4] Laughter is good medicine, the saying goes. It is true. Laughter is good for our mental well-being because endorphins are released in our brains when we laugh. Do you need to spend time with children to learn to laugh?

Develop some "delightful diversions." One of my mentors, Dr. Tim Ruden, calls hobbies "delightful diversions." He said, "God uses them to help us detach from stress and attach to His joy." He recommends that we make a list of potential hobbies and experiment with them.

As you try those activities, ask, "Is this replenishing my spirit?" I remember reading once that you relax with your hands if you work with your brain. Knowledge workers often relax through hands-on hobbies—gardening, carpentry, or sports. In addition, if you work with your hands, you relax through your brain. People who have physically taxing jobs often relax through reading, writing, or contemplating. Consider this principle when choosing your hobbies.

Create a life-giving list. As you journey through life, pay attention to the activities that fill your emotional bucket and the ones that drain your bucket. The activities that fill you up belong on your "life-giving" list. Proactively carve out time for them in your busy schedule. Don't hope for time; make time. Set the goal of incorporating one or two of these into your life every day. In addition, seek to balance activities that drain you with activities that are life-giving. If your day is filled with meetings and meetings drain you, proactively carve out some time for what fills you. You may carve out ten minutes in between meetings to go for a brisk walk in the sunshine.

Perhaps music is on your life-giving list. If so, proactively schedule a time to enjoy it because, in the words of Sally Morgenthaler, "Music has the ability to access the human soul faster than anything else. . . . Our whole society—especially those younger than 30—craves the medicine of music."[5] Take your medicine—the medicine of music!

Leverage time off and vacations. Rest helps you be at your best.

> The business world is often suspicious of retreats, perhaps in part because of the word's military meaning: moving backward and possibly giving up. But for the aware leader, the long-distance winner, stepping back is anything but a defeat; it's a chance to gather new energy and ideas for the next campaign.[6]

If you have time off, use it to gather new energy and ideas. If you feel guilty when you take time off, perhaps you are wrestling with the messiah complex. Leighton Ford, in *Transforming Leadership*, explains:

> Sometimes we think that God's work depends so much on us that we become feverish, compulsive and overly involved—workaholics of the kingdom rather than disciples of the King. This kind of hyperactivism does not come from the obedience of faith but from the anxiety of unbelief. Fearful that if we do not "go, go, go," our plans—or even God's cause—will fail, we get into a kind of messiah complex, believing that it is up to us to save the world. And so we end up burned out.[7]

Have a weekly Sabbath. "Remember the Sabbath day by keeping it holy" (Exodus 20:8). God commanded the Israelites to practice the Sabbath, giving them a day every week to play and pray.

"What would I do on a Sabbath?" you wonder.

Patrick Klingaman recommends you ask two questions to have a meaningful Sabbath:

- Will this activity help me turn my attention and focus to God?
- Will this activity help me become more rested and refreshed?[8]

Rest and worship are the two key ingredients of a meaningful Sabbath.

Rest restores our physical vitality and renews our emotional energies. In restful solitude, we forget the world with its pressing demands for a while and remember who we are. Worship goes a step farther and enables us to forget ourselves for a while and remember Who God is. It puts everything into perspective. In worship we remember the goodness and the greatness of God.[9]

Balancing the Two Modes

In his helpful book *Clergy Self-Care*, Roy Oswald writes about the two modes of life. The first mode is what he called "intra-dependence." The following words characterize this:

Doing

Working

Role

Responsibility

Achievement

The second mode, according to Oswald, is called "extra-dependence," which is characterized by the following words:

Being

Play

Essence

Sabbath time

Grace

We need to spend time in both modes to live a healthy, balanced life.[10]

May God help you to balance working hard with playing hard . . . and laughing hard!

BEYOND THE BOOK

Takeaway: Be ambitious at both work *and* play.

Verse to memorize: "Teach those who are rich in this world not to be proud and not to trust in their money, which is so unreliable. Their trust should be in God, who richly gives us all we need for our enjoyment" (1 Timothy 6:17 NLT).

Questions to consider: What activities would I put on my life-giving list? How can I make time for more of these activities?

Reflections: _____

_____

_____

_____

_____

_____

Prayer: *Lord, I feel guilty when I play. Please release me from that guilt, knowing that there is a time to work and a time to play. Help me to find the balance. Lead me to discover some delightful* *diversions that help me detach from stress and attach to You and those I love. By faith, I chose to become ambitious about having fun. Amen.*

Application: Do a hobby experiment. Make a list of five hobbies and try them. As you do them, notice if they are life-giving or not.

CHAPTER TWENTY

The Myths About Medication

Then Isaiah said, "Prepare a poultice of figs." They did so and applied it to the boil, and he recovered.

2 Kings 20:7

He trained and equipped pastors for many years. I met with him to get some advice on a few challenges I faced. As we sat at our restaurant table, I heard the chatter of people talking behind me. I smelled the delicious aroma of bacon sizzling on the grill in the kitchen.

"Pastors go through many challenges and difficulties. Many are depressed and discouraged," he said. "I have suffered with depression myself and know how difficult it is."

I took a sip of coffee and nodded my head in agreement. *Been there*, I thought.

"I wish more pastors would take medication for their depression. But they won't for fear of being labeled spiritually weak."

"I couldn't agree more," I said. As he said those words I thought, *I wish more believers could hear his words*. Perhaps they will hear them through this book.

Can you relate to his words? Are you avoiding medication because you don't want to be labeled as weak? Do you believe taking medicines for depression or any other mental illness shows a lack of faith? If so, ponder these four truths.

Humans Are Multifaceted

We are composed of body, soul, and spirit. "Now may the God of peace himself sanctify you completely, and may your whole spirit and soul and body be kept blameless at the coming of our Lord Jesus Christ" (1 Thessalonians 5:23 ESV). The central theme of this book is that if we want to achieve a higher level of mental well-being, we need to take a multifaceted approach. We need to leverage the four keys—spiritual, mental, physical, and relational—not just one or two.

If someone had come to me twenty-five years ago and shared their struggle with mental illness, I would have responded by saying, "You need to pray about it. You need to read the Bible more." I would have left out the other three keys. Are prayer and Bible study important? Of course! Yet we also need to include the other three areas.

One of the areas I have witnessed well-meaning Christians leave out is the biological one. They fail to realize that at the root of their mental illness is a biological source. To remedy it, they may need biological help like medication.

You say, "I am waiting for God to heal me." I respect that. Please, however, allow me to push back for a moment by reminding you that God can heal you through natural *or* supernatural means, through miracles *or* medicine. Please be open to either way. They both come from our compassionate God.

Don't have double standards

If I take medication, I'm not trusting God. If I use medication, my faith is weak. Are thoughts like those running through your mind? If so, consider the counterargument I heard once.

"Do you eat food? Do you drink water?"

"Of course," the person declared.

"Why do you eat food? Why do you drink water? Why don't you have enough faith to believe that God will provide you with hydration and calories?"

Just as we need food for nutrition and water for hydration, we may need medicine for our biological and chemical needs.

Research has concluded that neurotransmitters in the brain are reduced in clinically depressed individuals. Serotonin, one of these neurotransmitters, is a chemical courier that connects individual brain cells so that thoughts and emotions can occur normally. Prescription antidepressants attempt to repair the chemical imbalance that causes depression. Certain medications aid in restoring balance and allow serotonin to gradually replenish itself.[1]

Consider the Bible

Are you aware that there are numerous times in the Bible when people used medication for healing? For example:

HEZEKIAH

"In those days Hezekiah became ill and was at the point of death" (2 Kings 20:1). Hezekiah was the thirteenth king of Judah. One day, he became deathly ill. So he prayed to God and asked for His help. God answered his prayers and gave the prophet Isaiah a message to deliver to him. "Prepare a poultice of figs" (2 Kings 20:7).

A poultice of figs was a hot, soft mass of figs and other ingredients commonly used in ancient times to treat skin infections. The prophet Isaiah instructed Hezekiah to use medicine for healing. What was the result? "They did so and applied it to the boil, and he recovered" (2 Kings 20:7). Is it possible that God wants to bring you to a new level of health through medication?

THE GOOD SAMARITAN

A Jewish man walked the seventeen-mile journey from Jerusalem to Jericho. As he looked at the steep cliffs and rough terrain, perfect places for thieves to hide, he might have prayed, "God, protect me from bandits and thieves."

Tragically, he was attacked by bandits and left for dead on the side of the road. While two religious people passed by him without helping, the most unlikely person stopped and helped—a hated Samaritan. "He took pity on him. He went to him and bandaged his wounds, *pouring on oil and wine*" (Luke 10:33–34, emphasis added).

Why did the Samaritan pour oil and wine on the man? Those were ancient forms of medicine. Next, he put the man on his donkey and took him to an inn. The Samaritan, the hero of the story, used medication to help the man recover from his injuries.

THE MEDICINE OF SPIT

"He took the blind man by the hand and led him outside the village. When he had spit on the man's eyes and put his hands on him, Jesus asked, 'Do you see anything?'" (Mark 8:23).

Why did Jesus spit on the man's eyes? "Several Roman writers and Jewish rabbis considered saliva to be a valid treatment for blindness."[2] In other words, in the ancient world, people believed that saliva had medicinal qualities. Jesus used a medicine of the day to heal the man.

Trust Jehovah-Rapha

One of the Hebrew names for God is Jehovah-Rapha, which means, "the Lord who heals." God is a healer. As the sovereign healer, He can heal through supernatural means—through faith and prayer. He can also heal through natural means, like doctors and medication. Are you open to both ways?

Practical Steps

If a doctor has prescribed you medication for your mental well-being, let me make a few suggestions:

Be patient. You won't feel better right away. It takes time for the medication to kick in. I was made aware of this the first time a doctor prescribed medication for my mental well-being.

"How long will it take to kick in?" I asked, hoping for quick relief.

My hopes for a quick fix were dashed when he said, "It could take as long as six weeks for you to notice any changes."

"Six weeks," I said. "I don't know if I can make it through today."

God's grace got me through that dark time. When the medicine kicked in, I felt better. It didn't happen overnight, but it did over time.

Be Consistent. Figure out a system that will help you be consistent in taking your medicine. Perhaps you will use one of those pill organizers and set a reminder on your phone. Consistency is key when it comes to taking your medication.

Check with your doctor before you stop taking your medications. Don't ever stop taking your medication without the guidance of your doctor. One of the common mistakes people make is to quit their medication if they feel better. Don't do it. Consult your doctor before you make a change in your medication.

Lying on the Floor Between Services

During a time in which I was struggling with the stigma of taking medication, I decided to do the opposite of what I just shared with you. I decided to go off my depression medication without consulting my doctor. This caught up to me one Sunday morning.

Sunday mornings are a highlight of my week. I deeply enjoy serving the Lord by loving people and gracefully delivering His truth to the flock. During this season of our church's ministry, we had three Sunday morning worship services. Doing three services was very taxing and draining.

As a result of going off my medication, I remember feeling lifeless and dull. I could sense that my brain was not functioning properly—like an engine misfiring. I ended up lying on the floor in between services in my office. *God, help me get through this day*, I prayed.

Thankfully, God gave me the power to make it through that Sunday, and no one knew what I was struggling with. I began taking my medication again the next day.

————— **BEYOND THE BOOK** —————

Takeaway: God is a healer and may choose to heal you naturally or supernaturally!

Verse to memorize: "Then Isaiah said, 'Prepare a poultice of figs.' They did so and applied it to the boil, and he recovered" (2 Kings 20:7).

Questions to consider: Do you have a stigma against taking medication for mental illness? Why or why not?

Reflections: _____

_____

_____

_____

_____

Prayer: *Lord, You are my healer. I acknowledge that You have many healing tools at Your disposal. You can heal me supernaturally through faith and prayer or naturally through doctors and medicine. I am open to either way. Please give me the humility to take medication if that is what I need to feel better. Give me patience to find the right medication and the persistence to stick with it until it begins to work in my body. Amen.*

Application: Read over the Bible stories I have shared in this chapter and ask God to speak to your heart. Notice that God uses medication to help people.

CHAPTER TWENTY-ONE

The Spirituality of Sleep

In peace I will lie down and sleep, for you alone, LORD, make me dwell in safety.

Psalm 4:8

Why are some teenagers happier than others? What do happy teens do that unhappy ones don't? An article in *Psychology Today* answers these questions. First, happier teens spend less time on their phones. They detach from technology. Second, they get enough sleep. "The strongest correlation with happiness is sleep—teens who say they get more than seven hours of sleep more nights are happier."[1]

Happy teens detach from technology and get enough sleep. What's valid for teens is also true for adults. Do you need to fast from technology? Are you controlling your screen time, or is it controlling you?

Moreover, are you getting enough sleep? Are you a good steward of your sleep? If not, you are not alone. I remember reading once that tired people run our world. Are you one of them?

Speaking from personal experience, when I don't sleep well, I don't feel well. My thoughts grow darker, my feelings feel colder, and my life seems harder. Lousy sleep puts a dark lens over my eyes, and I see the world despairingly. It makes me feel as though I'm walking uphill all day, and everything seems more challenging.

The opposite is true as well. When I get a good night's sleep, I feel as though I am walking downhill all day. Things seem more manageable. When I get my rest, I feel at my best. I see more clearly, think more deeply, and love more meaningfully.

"Sleep is sacred," a friend told once me. I agree. Do you grasp the importance of sleep to your overall health? Or are you taking it for granted?

The Benefits of Good Sleep

A good night's sleep is priceless. Ponder the benefits of good sleep:

- It regulates the release of essential hormones.
- It slows the aging process.
- It boosts our immune system.
- It improves brain function.
- It reduces cortisol levels.

Investing in a good night's sleep is one of the wisest investments you can make. It will pay enormous dividends in your mental well-being. In *How God Changes Your Brain*, we read:

> Sleep is so important to the brain that we cannot survive without it. Like other body parts, it needs time to rejuvenate and strengthen the connections between nerve cells. This process, called "consolidation," enables nerve cells to strengthen their connections. If the brain does not rest, those circuits will be damaged.[2]

The Spirituality of Sleep

After the triumphant victory on Mount Carmel, where God empowered Elijah to defeat the prophets of Baal, Elijah is threatened

156

by Jezebel and falls into a suicidal depression. He goes from the mountain top emotionally to the valley. How does he recover?

> Then he lay down under the bush and *fell asleep*. All at once an angel touched him and said, "Get up and eat." He looked around, and there by his head was some bread baked over hot coals, and a jar of water. He ate and drank and *then lay down again*. The angel of the LORD came back a second time and touched him and said, "Get up and eat, for the journey is too much for you."
>
> 1 Kings 19:5–7, emphasis added

Did you see the references to him resting and sleeping? Perhaps there is a lesson here. If we are mentally dark, we may need to catch up on our sleep. Here are four ways to do that:

Do a sleep audit. Would you consider doing a sleep audit? This is where you carve out time to evaluate the quality and quantity of your sleep. Try keeping a sleep journal in which you write down how much sleep you got, the quality of your sleep, and how you felt. In doing so, you will see the importance of a good night's sleep.

Develop a sleep routine. Being a teenager in the '90s, I admired Michael Jordan. I wanted to "Be Like Mike."[3] I copied several things from him, including his jersey number and free throw routine. Before most basketball players shoot a free throw, they go through their pre-free throw routine, which is the same action every time. Michael's free throw routine was that he spun the ball and bounced it three times. Then he would spin it again and bounce the ball twice, and then he would shoot. That is what I did (with much less success).

What if you developed a pre-bedtime routine like MJ's free throw routine? If you did the same things in the same order before bed, might that condition your brain to realize it's time to go to sleep and help you sleep better? Would you consider developing a pre-bedtime routine?

Perhaps you want to add some of the following ingredients to it:

- Don't look at a screen for an hour or two before bed.
- Don't drink water for at least four hours before bed.
- Get exercise during the day, which helps you sleep better at night.
- Have a wind-down time before bed.
- Process your stress before you lay down. (I will explain how to do that later.)
- Read Scripture before bed.
- Pray.
- Try to go to sleep and get up at the same time every day.
- Stop consuming caffeine at least six hours before bed.
- Make hard choices. You may have to make unpopular choices, dismissing yourself from a party early or saying no to watching that extra episode.
- If you have tried these things and are still not sleeping well, I recommend seeing a sleep expert.
- Use your bed for sleep and intimacy. Don't do work in it. Train your mind to see your bed as a place to rest, not work.

Process your stress before sleep. Have you ever laid down to sleep but your mind begins racing with a barrage of thoughts? *What if this happens? I forgot to do that. I am not sure how to handle that situation at work.* These racing thoughts remind me of a group of monkeys I once saw at the zoo, jumping from tree to tree. Our thoughts can be like those monkeys when we lay down to sleep. How do we tame those "thought monkeys?" The remedy is to block out some time before bed to process them, asking, *Lord, what do You want me to do about this? How should I view this?* You may also want to turn to the chapter "The Joy of Journaling" and do the "What's bothering me?" or the ABCDE exercises.

Don't wait to get into bed to process your "thought monkeys." Tame them before you lay under the covers lest they keep you awake all night. In addition, hand them to the Lord in prayer.

Be humble. As followers of Jesus, we strive to display the fruit of the Spirit in our lives. "But the fruit of the Spirit is love, joy, peace, forbearance, kindness, goodness, faithfulness, gentleness and self-control. Against such things there is no law" (Galatians 5:22–23).

One of the overlooked ways to display the fruit of the Spirit in our lives is to get enough sleep.

> I once struggled with the truth that patience is the fruit of the Holy Spirit because I knew from experience that it is also a fruit of a good night's rest. In other words, I was crabbier on little rest and less so on good rest. What brought light to this perplexity is that one of the ways the Spirit produces his fruit in our lives is by humbling us enough to believe that we are not God and that God can run the world without our staying up too late and getting up too early.[4]

Jesus Took Naps

Frank Boreham, a British pastor and author, dedicated his life to serving God. One of his practices was to take a nap for an hour every day.[5] Other famous nappers were John F. Kennedy, Ronald Reagan, Thomas Edison, Winston Churchill, and Jesus.

"Jesus was in the stern, sleeping on a cushion. The disciples woke him and said to him, 'Teacher, don't you care if we drown?'" (Mark 4:38). If Jesus needed sleep, so do we. May you ask God to help you become a wise steward of your sleep! As you lay your head to sleep, remind yourself that the world is in good hands—it's in God's hands.

BEYOND THE BOOK

Takeaway: Be a wise steward of your sleep.

Verse to memorize: "I lie down and sleep; I wake again, because the LORD sustains me" (Psalm 3:5).

Question to consider: What is my sleep routine?

Reflections:

Prayer: *"I lie down this night with God, and God will lie down with me; I lie down this night with Christ, and Christ will lie down with me; I lie down this night with the Spirit, and the Spirit will lie down with me; God and Christ in the Spirit be lying down with me."*[6]

Application: Do a sleep audit for seven days. Write down the following.

Date	Bedtime	Wake up time	The total amount of sleep	Rate the quality of your sleep: 1–10	Other notes:
1/10/25	9:00	5:00	8 hours	7	*I drank too much caffeine before bed. I will avoid it next time.*
1/11/25	9:30	5:30	8 hours	8	*I avoided the caffeine and slept much better.*

PART FOUR

The Relationship Key

The second is this: "Love your neighbor as yourself."

Mark 12:31

CHAPTER TWENTY-TWO

The Call of Connection

It is not good for the man to be alone.

Genesis 2:18

"Bear is so depressed," I said to my wife, Tammy.

Bear was our black-and-brown family dog. Being a mixture of German shepherd and golden retriever, he had both protective and friendly sides. His thick fur was soft to the touch. In many ways, I considered him the ideal dog.

Tammy agreed. "It's as if he is slowly dying of a broken heart."

Bear was lonely because his two companions—Cupcake, a severely obese beagle, and Brownie, a large black German shepherd had recently died. He grew up with them by his side. They were like the three musketeers. They did everything together. Now he was alone.

Before our eyes, we saw our lovely Bear slowly wilt away. He moped around our house like a limp sock—lifeless and forlorn. Sensing that he did not have much time left, Tammy came up with an idea. "What if we got two puppies that Bear could train before he dies?"

This suggestion was not new. We had discussed getting two puppies so that they could grow up together and keep each other company. I agreed, so we jumped in the car and headed for Wadena, Minnesota, to pick up these two flop-eared puppies. The kids later named them Brock and Bennett. They were a unique blend of bloodhound and bullmastiff. After paying for our new pups, we drove them back home. They slept most of the way.

How is Bear going to respond? I thought.

Something unexpected happened when we brought those puppies home—Bear came alive. He went from being down in the dumps to brimming with energy. It was as if getting those puppies gave him a renewed sense of purpose. It also gave him a furry family to which he could belong. As a result of getting Brock and Bennett, Bear lived three additional years. Much longer than we expected.

When Bear was alone, he was depressed. He came to life when he had a community around him. What's true for Bear is true of us. We need each other. Alone, we wither and die; together, we heal and thrive!

It Is Not Good for Man to Be Alone

Dr. Dean Ornish found that loneliness and isolation "increase the likelihood of disease and premature death *from all causes* by 200 to 500 percent or more. . . . Anything that promotes feelings of love and intimacy is healing; anything that promotes isolation, separation, loneliness . . . often leads to suffering, disease, and premature death."[1]

If you want to move toward greater mental well-being, you need to find your tribe, discover your people, and create a network of nurturing and loving relationships where you can love and be loved and care and be cared for.

You need to find your Brock and Bennet.

This is important because, "Great relationships lead to a significant increase in life satisfaction," wrote Tom Rath and Donald Clifton in *How Full is Your Bucket?* "Noted psychologist Ed

Diener found that 'The happiest people have high-quality social relationships.' On the other hand, Diener and other researchers have found that lonely people suffer psychologically."[2]

Satan understands your need for healthy connections. As a result, he works overtime to isolate you.

> Our generation longs for deep connection yet often settles for shallow ways of relating. In the wake of such high rates of divorce, neglect, and abuse, emerging generations long for connection, yet have been programmed for aloneness.[3]

Programmed for Aloneness?

Have you allowed Satan and our rugged, individualistic culture to program you for aloneness? Do you feel stranded on an island of isolation?

I came across a lonely soul one day as I read a comment card from Sunday's church attendance. So that we can be more effective, our church surveys new people. One of the questions we ask is, "What did you like best about your visit today?" We normally hear answers like, "The sermon," "The music," or "The kids' ministry." I looked in disbelief as I read this card. The person responded, "I felt love for the first time in two years."

There are many lonely people out there. Are you one of them?

My Lone Ranger Mindset

I am a recovering Lone Ranger. I tend to isolate myself. In fact, I am convinced that isolation was one of the contributing factors to my breakdown in 2002. This became clear to me in a meeting with two of my mentors, Jerry and Clarence. They had come down to try and talk me out of quitting the ministry.

"How are you doing?" one asked.

"I just don't know if I want to do this anymore. I think I am done with the ministry," I explained. The problems I was facing seemed too overwhelming. It seemed as if everything I did to make things better didn't help. I believed that my only option was to quit. As I shared my heart, I saw the concerned look on their faces.

"Please don't quit. Instead, I want to encourage you to take a three-month sabbatical. Wait until you are back from your sabbatical to make your decision," Clarence said. Next, he asked me a pivotal question. "Who are your friends in the ministry?"

I froze!

"I don't have any," I replied in disbelief. *I have fallen into the Lone Ranger trap,* I thought.

"In the future, you must prioritize connecting with other pastors. They will understand the pressure and challenges of pastoring."

I nodded in agreement. He then looked at Jerry and said something I have never forgotten.

He pointed at Jerry and said, "He is the most connected pastor I know." He then turned to me and said these painful yet true words, "You are the most disconnected pastor I know."

Ouch!

He was right! I had fallen into the Lone Ranger trap. Have you?

After I returned from my sabbatical, I made it a top priority to build relationships, especially with other pastors who could understand the pastoral reality.

Lone Ranger Christianity

Have you fallen into the trap of Lone Ranger living? Are you disconnected from life-giving relationships? I read once that in America we are rich in achievements but poor in relationships. This is not the biblical way. God created us to live life in a community of other believers.

> Two people are better off than one, for they can help each other succeed. If one person falls, the other can reach out and help. But someone who falls alone is in real trouble. Likewise, two people lying close together can keep each other warm. But how can one be warm alone? A person standing alone can be attacked and defeated,

but two can stand back-to-back and conquer. Three are even better, for a triple-braided cord is not easily broken.

Ecclesiastes 4:9–12 NLT

Solomon, the wisest man who ever lived, teaches that we were created to connect with others. Life is not a do-it-yourself project. It is wiser to live your life in a community of other people. Like Bear needed Brock and Bennet, we need each other.

We Were Created for Connection

Sue Johnson and Kenneth Sanderfer, in *Created for Connection*, write:

> We are created for connection. This drive to emotionally attach—to find someone to whom we can turn and say, "Hold me tight"—is wired into our mind, soul, and spirit. It is as basic to life, health, and happiness as the drives for food, shelter, and sex. We need emotional attachments with a few irreplaceable others to be physically and mentally healthy—to survive.[4]

Have you fully grasped the truth that to be healthy and whole, you need God and others? You were created to connect with God and others. It's in your divine DNA.

Frieda

Friedrich Stapel, a farmer from Germany, saw an unknown object as he was moving his herd of cows to a new pasture.

What's that? he thought as he walked toward it. As he got closer, he discovered that a wild boar piglet had joined his herd. And while he knew the damage wild boars could cause, he couldn't bring himself to chase the animal away.

He decided to adopt the piglet and name it Frieda. Knowing that local hunters might want to harm Frieda, he warned them to leave her alone.

Frieda became a local attraction. People came from all over to see this little pig who had been adopted into a herd of cows.[5]

In a similar way, if you have put your faith in Jesus Christ as your Lord and Savior, you have been adopted into God's family. "The Spirit you received does not make you slaves, so that you live in fear again; rather, the Spirit you received brought about your adoption to sonship. And by him we cry, 'Abba, Father'" (Romans 8:15).

As a member of God's family, I want to encourage you to prioritize building relationships with other believers. In *Celebration of Discipline*, Richard Foster quotes Isaac Pennington, who says that when people are gathered for genuine worship, "they are like a heap of fresh and burning coals warming one another as a great strength and freshness and vigor of life flows into all."[6]

Just as coal needs other coal to keep warm, we need each other. Admitting your need of others is not a sign of weakness; it's a sign of wisdom. Would you consider investing time in building healthy, tight-knit relationships with others?

Would you consider finding your Brock and Bennet? Like Bear, it may add years to your life!

BEYOND THE BOOK

Takeaway: You were created for connection. It is not good for you to be alone.

Verse to memorize: "Two people are better off than one, for they can help each other succeed" (Ecclesiastes 4:9 NLT).

Questions to consider: Do you have a Lone Ranger mindset? If so, where does this come from?

Reflections: _____

Prayer: *Lord, help me avoid the rut of rugged individualism. Remind me that You created me for connection, companionship, and collaboration. Show me a small group of people with whom I can build meaningful relationships. May those relationships serve as a safety net when I fall. By faith, I chose to prioritize the building of meaningful relationships. Amen.*

Application: Make a connection plan. Write out a list of people you are going to prioritize connecting with on a regular basis. In addition, explore some support groups. Look for a group with whom you can do life.

CHAPTER TWENTY-THREE

The Blessings of Boundaries

Do not move an ancient boundary stone set up by your ancestors.

Proverbs 22:28

The grass is greener in my neighbor's yard, I often think, as I stare at his manicured shrubs and green, lush lawn. I do my best to avoid the comparison game as I look at my unattended yard with its brown spots, uneven grass, and well-worn lawn chairs. I sometimes think, *Why can't my yard look like his?*

He might think, *I wish I could go into his lawn and spice it up. What is wrong with that guy? Why doesn't he take better care of his yard?*

My neighbor has never said anything like that to me, but it wouldn't surprise me if he thought it. In addition, he has never come into my yard and tried to spice it up (although I would be okay if he did).

He has never done this because of a basic rule of being a good neighbor is that you are responsible for your own yard. You are not responsible for your neighbor's yard. His yard is his responsibility; my yard is my responsibility.

A yard can teach us volumes about boundaries. Boundaries instruct that there are certain things we are responsible for and other things we are *not* responsible for. In this chapter, I want to share with you how to stay in your own yard. I want to teach you about boundaries. Before I do, I must credit Henry Cloud and John Townsend, bestselling authors and clinical psychologists. They have taught me most of what I know about boundaries. Dr. Cloud defines boundaries this way: "Boundaries, in short, define us. In the same way that a physical boundary defines where a property line begins and ends, a psychological and spiritual boundary defines who we are and who we are not."[1]

The Serenity Prayer that I referred to in a previous chapter is a prayer of boundaries. "God, grant me the serenity to accept what I cannot change, courage to change what I can, and wisdom to know the difference."[2]

In other words, God, grant me the serenity to accept what is not in my yard of responsibility, the courage to change what is in my yard of responsibility, and the wisdom to know the difference.

The Importance of Boundaries

One of my sin struggles is people pleasing. "Unhealthy people pleasing can be defined as the tendency to cater to others' preferences to the detriment of personal well-being."[3]

I have wrestled with the "disease to please" all my life. On one hand, this inclination has made me excel in certain aspects of pastoring. I am sensitive to others' needs, listen to them, and make them feel cared for.

One of the adverse effects of this sin struggle, however, is that I can lose my yard. If I am not careful, I can lose track of where I end and others begin. I can take responsibility for things that are not in my yard and lose track of the things that are. Because of this disposition, I often tell myself, "Steve, stay in your yard."

Stay in Your Yard

One person's heart's desires, will, emotions, thoughts, and intentions are separate and distinct from others'. "Each heart knows its own bitterness, and no one else can share its joy" (Proverbs 14:10).

Psychologists call this reality the differentiation of self. Healthy people realize they are separate and distinct from others, even though they may be in close relationships. My wife and I have a motto we try to live by: You do you, I'll do me, we'll be one big happy family. "You do you" means that you have your yard of responsibility. "I'll do me" means that I have my yard of responsibility. "We'll be one big happy family" signifies that we are on the same team, even though our yards of responsibility may differ. Frederick Buechner sums up the idea that people can be connected yet have separate yards of responsibility. "But a marriage made in heaven is one where they become more richly themselves together than the chances are either of them could ever have managed to become alone."[4]

Guard Your Heart

Since your heart belongs to you, you need to guard it. "Above all else, guard your heart, for everything you do flows from it" (Proverbs 4:23). One of the ways you protect your heart is by setting clear boundaries. "Boundaries are our way of protecting and safeguarding our souls. Boundaries are designed to keep the good in and the bad out."[5]

What boundaries do you need to establish to guard your heart? Perhaps you need to set some boundaries around your use of technology. Are you in control of your technology, or is it controlling you? In *The Tech Wise Family*, Andy Crouch recommends having Sabbaths from technology. This is where you turn off your device one hour per day, one day a week, and one week a year.[6] Do you need to schedule a tech Sabbath?

Self-Control, Not Others Control

"But the fruit of the Spirit is love, joy, peace, forbearance, kindness, goodness, faithfulness, gentleness and self-control" (Galatians 5:22–23). Notice that the fruit of the Spirit is self-control. It is not controlling others. We set boundaries not to control others but to protect what is within our yard. It's a way of practicing self-control. This is important because the only person you can change and control is yourself. Trying to change and control others is a waste of your time. Are you more focused on self-control or controlling others?

A small group I was a part of once was focused on controlling others rather than self-control.

"My spouse does not care about my needs. She is so selfish," said one of the members. Resentment was oozing from his words. As he said it, I looked around the rectangle table where ten to fifteen people had come to share their struggles and faith with each other. His comment sparked a barrage of finger-pointing.

"It's all my boyfriend's fault," said another woman in the group. You could see her face getting red as she thought about the actions of her partner. As we went around the table, most of the people engaged in yard-jumping. Instead of focusing on what they could control—their actions and attitudes—they focused on what they couldn't—the actions and reactions of others. This all changed when the group leader pointed out our error.

"We have just spent the last half hour focusing on what we have no control over—the choices of others," she said in utter frustration. "That is a waste of time. Let us instead focus on what we can control—ourselves. How could we have responded differently? How could we have had a different attitude?"

After heeding the leader's instruction, the tone of the whole group changed. We jumped back into our own yards. Staying in my yard is one of the most important lessons I have learned in moving toward greater mental health. When I am experiencing anxiety and stress, it is often because I am focused on things outside of my yard of control. "Get back in your yard," I tell myself. As I do, I feel more peaceful. Thomas à Kempis wrote, "First keep yourself at peace; then you can quiet others. The peaceful man is of more use than the great doctor . . . therefore first be zealous for yourself, and then you may be justly zealous for your neighbour."[7]

Three Boundary Attitudes

Gary Smalley defines three necessary attitudes toward boundaries:

- "I am fully responsible for my thoughts, beliefs, feelings, and behavior.
- "I am not responsible for your thoughts, beliefs, feelings, or behavior.
- "In a relationship I can influence—but not control—the thoughts, beliefs, feelings, and behavior of another."[8]

How could you adopt these attitudes as your own? Imagine repeating them daily to train yourself on what is within your yard and what is not.

Respecting Others' Boundaries

"Seldom set foot in your neighbor's house—too much of you, and they will hate you" (Proverbs 25:17). In this verse, Solomon teaches us to respect the boundaries of others. One of the traits of mature people is that they not only set their limits but also respect the boundaries of others. They may not like them or want them; however, they respect them. Love respects the boundary lines of others. Are you respecting other people's boundaries?

Chad's Story

"Mommy, this year, I want to make a Valentine's card for everyone in my class," Chad told his mom. Chad was a shy kid who often felt like a fish out of water because the only attention the other kids gave him was to bully him or make fun of him. He often walked the hallways of school by himself and sat alone at the lunch table feeling like an outsider looking in.

After Chad told his mom his plan, her heart sank. She thought, "The kids will make fun of him for these cards and hurt him even more."

Despite her reservations, she decided to help him make the cards. For a few weeks after school, they diligently worked on the cards until they were all finished.

Finally, the big day came. Chad brought the cards to school to hand out to his classmates. His mom stayed at home. She was a nervous wreck. She expected the kids to do what they always did—break Chad's heart with rejection and ridicule.

She heard the front door open. In came Chad, who said enthusiastically, "Not a one . . . not a one!"

Not one had accepted the cards, his mom thought with disdain. But what Chad then said was, "I didn't forget a one, not a single one!"[9]

Instead of focusing on what he couldn't control—the actions and reactions of others—Chad had focused on what he could control—his actions and behaviors. He stayed in his own yard instead of jumping into the yards of others' responsibility.

As you journey through your day today, push the pause button from time to time and ask yourself, "Whose yard am I in?"

BEYOND THE BOOK

Takeaway: Boundaries define what is within your yard of responsibility and what is not. Stay in your yard.

Verse to memorize: "Better a patient person than a warrior, one with self-control than one who takes a city" (Proverbs 16:32).

Questions to consider: What am I responsible for? What am I not responsible for?

Reflections: _____

_____

_____

_____

_____

_____

Prayer: *Lord, sometimes my boundary lines become fuzzy. I forget where I end and others begin. Help me define my boundaries. Show me what is and isn't my responsibility. Help me clearly and graciously articulate my boundaries to others. Help me respect their boundaries, as well. Amen.*

Application: Which of the three attitudes of boundaries do you truly believe in and live out?

Y or N: I am fully responsible for my thoughts, beliefs, feelings, and behavior.

Y or N: I am not responsible for others' thoughts, beliefs, feelings, or behavior.

Y or N: In a relationship, I can influence but not control the thoughts, beliefs, feelings, and behaviors of another.

CHAPTER TWENTY-FOUR

The Force of Family

When his family heard about this, they went to take charge of him, for they said, "He is out of his mind."

Mark 3:21

I grew up on a family farm in southeastern Minnesota. We lived in an old, two-story white farmhouse surrounded by trees, fields, and gravel roads. A quiet stream meandered through our back pasture. After finishing our chores, my brothers and I spent a lot of time outdoors building forts, fishing, and playing sports.

It was a happy childhood . . . until the accident happened.

In June 1976, my mom was mowing our yard on a green John Deere riding mower. In a hurry, she looked behind her, and as she did, my two-year-old brother crawled out in front of her. Tragically, she ran over the lower part of him.

Our lives would never be the same.

God gave my mom the supernatural strength to lift the mower off him. *He's not going to live,* she thought, as she called the neighbor to come and drive them to the hospital. As she waited for the neighbor, she wrapped my brother in bed sheets. He was bleeding profusely.

The good news is that we lived about thirty minutes away from one of the most outstanding hospitals in the world—the Mayo Clinic. They, with God's help, were able to save my brother's life.

That accident shaped me in many ways. First, it took a significant toll on my family financially because my brother ended up having around forty costly surgeries. As a result, finances were a constant stress. I picked up a fear of scarcity that I have battled my whole life. *We won't have enough,* I have often thought, even though God has always provided.

Next, my mom had to play the caregiver role for my brother who was recovering from this accident. She had to constantly wrap his leg, drive him to doctor appointments, and make sure he took his medication. While she was focused on caretaking my brother, my dad worked several jobs to provide for our family. Consequently, I didn't see them much. There were times I felt unseen and unheard.

Looking back now, I realize that my parents were doing the best they could in the difficult situation they faced. I am so proud of them for not giving up and for leaning on Jesus to get them through that tragic time. In my young, five-year-old brain, however, I felt left behind. Because of this, I have also wrestled with the fear of abandonment.

One of the blessings of this accident is that my parents chose to turn to God in their pain, not away from Him. As a result, my parents instilled in me a deep faith in Jesus. "We would have never made it without Jesus," my mom says to this day. They also modeled other wonderful characteristics for me like hard work, responsibility, teamwork, and self-discipline.

Train Up a Child

My brother's lawn mower accident was one of the most pivotal events in my life. It shaped me in many ways. What is true of me is true of you. Your family history has shaped you. Are you aware of how?

"Start children off on the way they should go, and even when they are old they will not turn from it" (Proverbs 22:6). Are you aware of how your family of origin affected you? Are you aware of the patterns and habits you learned from your childhood? If you take the time to reflect on them, you will see that some of them were healthy, while others were not. No family is perfect. A wise person asks what he wants to continue from his family of origin and what he wants to discontinue. "When I was a child, I talked like a child, I thought like a child, I reasoned like a child. When I became a man, I put the ways of childhood behind me" (1 Corinthians 13:11). What childhood ways do you need to let go of?

There Are No Perfect Families in the Bible

The Bible is filled with imperfect families and flawed, dysfunctional, and unhealthy people. A good example of an imperfect family is the family of David:

- David handed over the five nephews of his wife Michal to the Gibeonites to be killed. He did this because of Michal's dad, Saul. (see 2 Samuel 21:1–2, 7–9).
- David's firstborn son, Amnon, raped his half sister Tamar and was killed by Absalom (see 2 Samuel 13).
- Adonijah, David's fourth son, was executed by Solomon for trying to take his power (see 1 Kings 2:24–25).
- David's unnamed child with Bathsheba died as a punishment for David's adultery (see 2 Samuel 12:14).
- Solomon had a downfall later in life because he had so many wives (see 1 Kings 11:1–4; Ecclesiastes 2:8–11).[1]

And you thought your family had issues? Whenever you get down on yourself because of your imperfect family, recall David's. If God can use David and his family, He can use yours.

Jesus' family also had issues. His family thought he was crazy. "When his family heard about this, they went to take charge of him, for they said, 'He is out of his mind'" (Mark 3:21).

If you attempt to have a perfect family, you are trying to do something that is impossible. Show yourself and your family of origin grace as you ask, "What do I need to let go of from my family of origin?"

One Generation to the Next

Do you know that your family tree, followed back to the 1800s, has molded you?

> When the Bible uses the word family, it refers to our entire extended family over three to four generations. That means your family, in the biblical sense, includes all your brothers, sisters, uncles, aunts, grandparents, great-grandparents, great-uncles and aunts, and significant others going back to the mid-1800s![2]

Are you aware of the positive traits that were handed down to you? Are you aware of the toxic traits they handed down?

As you explore these pivotal questions, perhaps you will recognize some dysfunction in you that was handed down to you. If so, make it a goal of yours to become a transitional person. Develop the attitude of, "By faith, the dysfunction stops with me. I am not going to hand it down to my kids. The chain of dysfunction is broken in Jesus' name." This is so important because your choices today can have an impact on your family hundreds of years from now.

> I, the LORD your God, am a jealous God, punishing the children for the sin of the parents to the third and fourth generation of those who hate me, but showing love to a thousand generations of those who love me and keep my commandments.
>
> Exodus 20:5–6

Are you aware that your choices affect not just you but the generations that come after you?

Mental Illness and Families

One of the predispositions that can run in families is mental illness. I was told by a mental health professional that we need to look at a person's family history, because mental illness often runs in families. In other words, just as certain physical illnesses can run in families, so can mental illness.

If you are wrestling with mental illness, this could be something that was passed down to you from your ancestors.

> A family history of depression does, however, appear to increase your risk. This has been documented in numerous studies examining depression in families. The findings show that first degree relatives—parents, siblings, children—of a depressed person have a higher risk of depression than do individuals without a family history of depression. The increase in risk may be related to genetics, family environment or both.[3]

In addition, you are more likely to wrestle with depression if you have experienced certain traumatic events in your life, such as these examples:

- Death of a parent or sibling
- Abandonment
- Neglect
- Physical or sexual abuse
- Chronic illness
- Traumatic event[4]

The Family of God

In this chapter, we have talked about how our family of origin shapes us. As followers of Jesus, we are also a part of the family of God. When you put your faith in Jesus as leader and forgiver, you become a son or daughter of God (see John 1:12–13). As a child of God, you become a member of God's family (see Ephesians 2:19). Andy Crouch writes:

The first family for everyone who wants wisdom and courage in the way of Jesus is the church—the community of disciples who are looking to Jesus to reshape their understanding and their character. And the church is, and can be, family for everyone in a way that biological families cannot. No matter whether your parents are still living—or whether they were ever loving—no matter whether you have a spouse or children or siblings or cousins, you have a family in the church.[5]

Spiritual growth is letting go of your past dysfunctional behaviors and adopting your new family's healthy behaviors. It's matching your attitude and behaviors to your new family's way of doing things—the family of God.

My Brother

Miraculously, my brother Josh, who was run over by the lawn mower, is a very athletic man today. You would never know he had so many surgeries. He has the energy of the Energizer Bunny. I often have a hard time keeping up with him.

BEYOND THE BOOK

Takeaway: There are no perfect families in the Bible.

Verse to memorize: "When I was a child, I talked like a child, I thought like a child, I reasoned like a child. When I became a man, I put the ways of childhood behind me" (1 Corinthians 13:11).

Questions to consider: What things do I want to carry forward from my family of origin? What do I want to leave behind?

Reflections:

Prayer: *Lord, thank You that there are no perfect families in the Bible. My family is far from perfect. Please help me to let go of the unhealthy attitudes and behaviors I learned from my family of origin so that I can live in alignment with my new family of God. By faith, from this day forward, I chose to live as a son or daughter of my heavenly Father. Amen.*

Application: Thank God for your family, no matter how imperfect it is. Joey Reiman says that if you have a loving family, you are a "famillionaire."[6] You wouldn't trade all the money in the world for it.

CHAPTER TWENTY-FIVE

The Elements of Empathy

For we do not have a high priest who is unable to empathize with our weaknesses, but we have one who has been tempted in every way, just as we are—yet he did not sin.

Hebrews 4:15

"Do you want me to come in with you?" the large man asked his friend. He looked at me with stern eyes and had his chest puffed out. He had joined his friend who had come to meet with me because he was angry over a decision I had made.

"No. I will speak to Pastor Steve by myself."

I felt a sense of relief.

"I will wait outside the door," the big man said as he slammed the door.

"What is bothering you?" I asked.

Up in arms, he shared his complaint with me for about an hour. By God's grace, I actively listened to him and showed empathy. I didn't try to out-argue him, nor did I try to show him why I was right and he was wrong. I listened to him and showed empathy.

"If I understand you, you feel [fill in the blank]. Is that accurate?" After actively listening and showing empathy, I asked if he felt understood.

"Yes," he replied. I could sense a shift in his spirit. He started smiling at me and unfolded his arms.

"Are you open to hearing my view on the situation?" I asked.

"Yes."

I explained my view, and afterward, he said something that shocked me.

"Pastor Steve, I knew that if you made that decision, it was the right one."

You were ready to tear my head off an hour ago, I thought. *Now you are praising me?*

That experience taught me a crucial lesson about forging healthy relationships: empathize and then explain. Before you explain your view on an issue, take the time to listen, understand, and empathize with the other person's view.

What Is Empathy?

The word *empathy* comes from the Greek words *in* and *feeling.* Empathy is being "in the feeling of the other." The apostle Paul encouraged empathy by writing, "Rejoice with those who rejoice; mourn with those who mourn" (Romans 12:15). He instructs us to enter into the feelings of another. If they are rejoicing, rejoice. If they are mourning, mourn.

Instead of trying to change another's feelings, empathize with them. The opposite of empathy is described in one of Solomon's proverbs. "Like one who takes away a garment on a cold day, or like vinegar poured on a wound, is one who sings songs to a heavy heart" (Proverbs 25:20). When someone has a heavy heart, don't sing songs of joy to them—empathize with them. Ask Jesus to shine His empathetic light through you.

The Empathy of Jesus

In the beginning was the Word, and the Word was with God, and the Word was God. He was with God in the beginning. Through him all things were made; without him nothing was made that has been made.

John 1:1–3

Note the word *Word*. To whom is that referring? From the text, we know that the Word was God. We learn something fundamental about the Word in verse 14:

> The Word became flesh and made his dwelling among us. We have seen his glory, the glory of the one and only Son, who came from the Father, full of grace and truth.
>
> John 1:14

The Word—God—became flesh and made His dwelling among us. God moved into our neighborhood. We celebrate this every year at Christmas. Who is the Word? Jesus. Why did He move into our neighborhood? One reason was to show us empathy.

> For we do not have a high priest who is unable to *empathize with our weaknesses*, but we have one who has been tempted in every way, just as we are—yet he did not sin. Let us then approach God's throne of grace with confidence, so that we may receive mercy and find grace to help us in our time of need.
>
> Hebrews 4:15–16, emphasis added

Because Jesus walked a mile in our moccasins, He can empathize with our weaknesses, trials, struggles, and pain. As His followers, we are to model our lives after Him. One way we do that is by showing empathy to others. "Finally, all of you, be likeminded, be sympathetic, love one another, be compassionate and humble" (1 Peter 3:8).

Seek First to Understand

Years ago, I came across a statement by Stephen Covey that had a deep impact on me regarding healthy relationships: Seek first to understand, then to be understood. Covey explains:

> "Seek first to understand" involves a very deep shift in paradigm. We typically seek first to be understood. Most people do not listen

with the intent to understand; they listen with the intent to reply. They're either speaking or preparing to speak. They're filtering everything through their own paradigms, reading their autobiography into other people's lives.[1]

Simply put, listen first and talk second. In the book of James, God shares the correct sequence for healthy communication. "My dear brothers and sisters, take note of this: Everyone should be quick to listen, slow to speak and slow to become angry" (James 1:19). Many people have the wrong sequence. They are quick to talk and be angry, but they are slow to listen—if they really listen at all.

When it comes to good listening, I recommend the three R's:

Restate Content. After listening to another's view, restate what you heard in your own words. "If I understand you correctly, you said . . . Is that accurate?" Note how I checked in to make sure I understood the other person's view. This is important because it is easy to assume we understand another person when we don't.

Reflect feeling. Don't just listen to the content of their message; listen for the emotions behind the message. This is important because:

> True communication usually does not occur until each person understands the feelings that underlie the spoken words. People generally feel more understood, cared for, and connected when the communication focuses on their emotions and feelings rather than merely on their words or thoughts.[2]

After you have identified their emotion, name it. "You seem frustrated."

Render empathy. Next, express empathy to the person by saying something like one of these:

- "I can see how that would be difficult for you."
- "I understand why you would feel that way."
- "That must be frustrating."

- "It's completely normal to feel that way in this situation."
- "I can only imagine how challenging this has been for you."
- "Your feelings are valid, and it's okay to express them."
- "I appreciate you sharing this with me."
- "You're not alone in this; I'm here to support you."

Showing empathy does not mean you agree with the other person's view. Rather, it shows that you value them enough to listen to their thoughts on a subject. After the person feels listened to and understood, share your thoughts using "I" statements—"I feel . . . ," "I think . . ."

FBI Hostage Negotiator

In 1993, the Bureau of Alcohol, Tobacco, Firearms and Explosives raided a religious compound in Waco, Texas, because they believed the Branch Davidians were illegally stockpiling weapons and abusing children. The leader of the group was a self-proclaimed messiah named David Koresh. A fifty-one-day standoff ensued, and tragically, eighty people lost their lives.

Gary Noesner was the FBI's chief negotiator during much of that standoff. Under his leadership, thirty people came out of the compound alive; however, the higher-ups didn't think he was moving fast enough, so they replaced him. After he was replaced, no one else came out.

During his career, Noesner worked in many highly volatile situations like Waco. What was his approach in dealing with such dangerous situations? How did he bring peace in such a chaotic time? He followed something called the "behavioral change stairway." He describes the stairway this way:

> You listen to show interest, then respond empathetically, which leads to rapport building, which then leads to influence. But influence does not accrue automatically. We can suggest alternatives to violence, but we must first earn the right to be of influence.[3]

Ponder the four steps of the behavioral change stairway:

- *Active listening.* When Noesner faced emotionally charged situations, his first action was to listen to other people and make them feel heard. He asked open-ended questions. He led by listening, not defending.
- *Show empathy.* As he listened, he showed empathy. "I could see why you are upset." "You don't deserve this." "It's not fair."
- *Build trust.* As he actively listened and expressed empathy, something magical happened—the person began to trust him. Trust is built through an empathetic ear, not a dictatorial mouth.
- *Influence.* Once trust was built, he could influence and collaborate with the person. He went from an us-versus-them mindset to a *we* mindset, from a combative relationship to a collaborative one.

Would you consider trying his four steps if you have a strained relationship? Would you approach the situation with a big ear, not a big mouth? Would you consider expressing empathy, not anger?

BEYOND THE BOOK

Takeaway: Empathize, then explain.

Verse to memorize: "Fools find no pleasure in understanding but delight in airing their own opinions" (Proverbs 18:2).

Questions to consider: Am I quick to listen or quick to speak? Why?

Reflections:

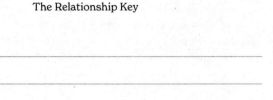

Prayer: *Lord, thank You for giving me two ears and one mouth. Please help me to use them accordingly. I admit that I am often quick to speak, defend, and argue. Change my ways, Lord. Help me to listen first and speak second. Please help me make others feel deeply heard and understood, even if I disagree. Amen.*

Application: Pick someone with whom you can practice good listening today. Tell them that you are seeking to improve your listening skills and ask them if they would be willing to role-play with you. As they share, remember the three R's:

- Restate content.
- Reflect feeling.
- Render empathy.

CHAPTER TWENTY-SIX

The Freedom of Forgiveness

"Father, forgive them, for they do not know what they are doing."

Luke 23:34

My family loves animals—especially dogs. When we get together for family gatherings, we often spend most of the time talking about the animals. "Remember when Cupcake did this? Do you remember when Bear did that?" Two of our dogs used to get into heated conflicts: Cupcake and Brownie.

Cupcake was our severely obese beagle. Her head looked normal, but her body looked as though she had swallowed a barrel. "Now I know why you call her Cupcake," a visitor chuckled when they saw her for the first time. "I can see she has eaten a lot of cupcakes." In addition, Cupcake was as stubborn as a mule and had a laser-like focus on food. She lived to eat.

Brownie was the alpha dog of the house. She ruled the roost. She was a large, black German shepherd with a strong protective side. Most people and other dogs were intimidated by her.

Not Cupcake!

Cupcake liked to challenge Brownie's authority, especially when it came to food. If Brownie had some food, for example, Cupcake would get in her face and try to take it. Brownie was patient with her. She would give her some warnings by assertively showing her razor like teeth, communicating "Back off. Leave my food alone." Cupcake would not listen. After several warnings, Brownie would snap at Cupcake, often leaving her bleeding and hurt.

I know the two dogs loved each other. When they went to the dog park, they were like macaroni and cheese; you couldn't separate them. Even though they loved each other, they would hurt and wound each other.

What's true for dogs is true for humans: We hurt and wound one another. The question is not if we will be hurt by others—that's a given. The real question is whether or not we will we forgive those who have hurt us.

In this chapter, I want to discuss the importance of forgiveness. Forgiveness is essential if you want to live the abundant life Jesus promised (John 10:10). It is also mandatory for your mental well-being. Simply put, unforgiveness leads to disease, whereas forgiveness leads to health.

Forgiveness Is . . .

What is forgiveness? The word *forgiveness* means to "send away." Instead of holding on to your hurt—replaying the cruel behavior in your mind, reviewing the oppressive situation in the shower, reliving the stinging pain on your drive to work—you release it into the healing hands of God.

Gary Neal Hansen defines forgiveness this way: "Forgiveness is when you've been harmed, but you actively, prayerfully lift the sentence and decide not to exercise your right to prosecute or avenge."[1]

Why Do We Forgive?

"Why should I forgive that person?" you protest. "They don't deserve it."

I agree. As followers of Jesus, however, we forgive others not because they deserve it. We forgive because Jesus tells us to, out of obedience to Jesus, and because He forgave us.

> Be kind and compassionate to one another, forgiving each other, just as in Christ God forgave you" (Ephesians 4:32).

> Bear with each other and forgive one another if any of you has a grievance against someone. Forgive as the Lord forgave you" (Colossians 3:13).

The foundation of forgiving others is God's forgiveness for us. Did we deserve to be forgiven by Jesus? I know I didn't. I am assuming you didn't as well. None of us are perfect. Yet he forgave us if we asked Him to (see 1 John 1:9).

As forgiven people, we need to be forgiving people. We need to ask Jesus to empower us to follow His example and forgive others as He forgave us.

Forgiveness Is a Choice

Every day, we have a choice. Will we forgive those who have hurt us or grow in resentment? What will you choose?

Years ago, I came across a helpful formula for responding wisely to the hurtful situations of life: E + R = O.[2] The E stands for the event or what happened to you. The R stands for your response. The O stands for the outcome. Healthy people focus on the R. In other words, they realize they often cannot control the E. They can, however, control their response to it. They know that their response is their responsibility. More than anything else, their response will determine the outcome of the event.

Forgiveness is focusing on the R. It's declaring, "It hurt. It mattered. I choose to let go and let God settle the score. I choose to focus on my dreams and goals, not these scars and wounds."

Unforgiveness Infects Others

"Watch out that no poisonous root of bitterness grows up to trouble you, corrupting many" (Hebrews 12:15 NLT). What happens when someone encounters you and your heart is overflowing with unforgiveness? Your unforgiveness spills over onto them. Your choice not to forgive someone doesn't just have an impact on you—it affects those with whom you do life. You've probably encountered people who have chips on their shoulders. They are nursing a grudge against someone. Their toxic spirit can infect an entire room. Are you such a person? Is the poison of unforgiveness flowing through your veins corrupting many?

Forgiveness and Trust Are Not the Same Thing

"Are forgiveness and trust the same thing?" you ask. No.

Forgiveness is a gift. Examine the word: For-*give*. Within the word *forgive* is the word *give*. Forgiveness is not something the other person earned. If that were the case, it would not be a gift. Forgiveness is a gift that you give to others and yourself.

On the other hand, trust is earned. Trust is earned through trustworthy behavior. You can forgive someone in a moment, but trust is earned over time by consistent character. "By their fruit you will recognize them" (Matthew 7:16). You earn trust by displaying trustworthy character (fruit) consistently over the long run. Often, building trust takes a long time.

The Steps of Forgiveness

"How do I forgive that person?" you might ask. Here are four steps to forgiveness.

Surrender your right to settle the score. We live in a culture that scripts us to seek revenge. "If someone has hurt us, hurt them back," we are taught. God teaches another way.

Do not take revenge, my dear friends, but leave room for God's wrath, for it is written: "It is mine to avenge; I will repay," says the Lord. On the contrary: "If your enemy is hungry, feed him; if he is thirsty, give him something to drink. In doing this, you will heap burning coals on his head." Do not be overcome by evil, but overcome evil with good.

Romans 12:19–21

Note carefully that phrase "leave room for God's wrath." When someone has hurt us, we can choose to let God settle the score, or we can seek to do it ourselves. The way to allow God to settle the score is to send that balloon of hurt to heaven. Put it in His hands.

Understand the person who hurt you. One Sunday morning, a church member made a comment I have never forgotten. "When someone hurts you," she said, "don't ask 'What's wrong with them?' But instead ask, 'What happened to them?'"

Every life is a story. Understanding a person's story can help you comprehend why they did what they did. They may be reacting to the trauma and difficulties they have experienced in life.

Please do not misunderstand me. I am not making excuses for their wrong behavior. I am simply saying that understanding other people's stories can help us understand the *why* behind their *what*.

Pray for your enemies. One of the best ways to forgive someone is to pray for them. "But I tell you, love your enemies and pray for those who persecute you" (Matthew 5:44). Notice that we are to love and pray for our enemies. Consider praying this prayer over that person you need to forgive: *Lord, I bless them. I forgive them and wish them well.*

Do good to them. Don't just pray for your enemies—bless them. "Love your enemies, do good to those who hate you, bless those who curse you, pray for those who mistreat you" (Luke 6:27–28).

One Sunday morning, I taught on Jesus' command to love our enemies. Afterward, I spoke with an elderly woman about the sermon. She had visited our church with a family member. As I spoke with her, I could sense her non-anxious presence. It brought me comfort. She had gray hair and a kind, gentle spirit. In those few moments of visiting, she said something I have never forgotten.

"My late husband, a pastor, had a unique way of loving his enemies. Guess what he did when someone from church went out of their way to hurt him?"

"Cut them out of his life. Stayed away from them?"

"No. He would bring them a pie."

Her husband modeled Jesus' command to love our enemies and do good to those who have hurt us. What if you followed his example? To whom do you need to bring a pie?

BEYOND THE BOOK

Takeaway: Forgiveness is a choice to send the pain away into God's hands. It's trusting God to settle the score. We forgive because Jesus forgave us.

Verse to memorize: "Bear with each other and forgive one another if any of you has a grievance against someone. Forgive as the Lord forgave you" (Colossians 3:13).

Question to consider: Do you understand the difference between forgiveness and trust? Forgiveness is a gift. Trust is earned.

Reflections:

Prayer: *Lord, I am hurt because* _____. *Please give me the ability to forgive* _____. *What they did hurt me. It was wrong. I am choosing, however, to leave room for Your wrath. I've decided to let you settle the score. Please help me to forgive them as You have forgiven me. Amen.*

Application: When you feel hurt because of another person's actions, pray this prayer over them: *Lord, I forgive them, I bless them, and I wish them well.* You may pray this prayer twenty times a day. Pray it in faith.

CHAPTER TWENTY-SEVEN

The Guidance of the Golden Rule

Be kind and compassionate to one another.

Ephesians 4:32

"How should I respond to that nasty email? How do I patch things up with that disgruntled family member? How can I help my friend get through this difficult time?"

Every day, we make choices about how we treat people. As followers of Jesus, love is to be our guide. "Love your neighbor as yourself" (Matthew 22:39). Jesus wanted His followers to be known for their love (see John 13:34).

Imagine having a tool in your pocket that would help you discern the loving way to treat another. Imagine if this tool was like a relational compass, guiding you on how to treat that cantankerous neighbor, annoying spam caller, or belligerent coworker. What is this relational compass?

The Golden Rule!

"So in everything, do to others what you would have them do to you, for this sums up the Law and the Prophets" (Matthew

7:12). The Golden Rule instructs us to treat others the way we would want to be treated. To do for others what we would want done to us.

Imagine seeing the Golden Rule as a compass for how you treat people. Before you acted or reacted to another person, what if you pushed the pause button and pondered, "If I were in their shoes, how would I want to be treated?" Thus, you treat them based on the Golden Rule, not your temporary mood or inclinations.

When I am having a grim, gloomy day, my feelings often instruct me to treat people poorly. If I am under a cloud of depression, my feelings cry, "Avoid them." If I am angry, my feelings shout, "Snap at them." If I am anxious, my feelings whisper, "Be suspicious of them." When I am out of sorts, thoughts like these enter my mind. During those moments, I choose to acknowledge those thoughts and feelings. "I am feeling heavy-hearted. Angry. Scared." Often, I write them down in a notebook. Either way, I ask the Lord to help me not act upon them. After Abraham Lincoln passed away, they found letters he had written to his generals in his desk, voicing his frustrations with them.[1] He never sent those letters. He used the process of writing down his feelings to clear his mind and spirit.

After acknowledging your feelings, pull out the Golden Rule compass and ask, "If I were in that person's shoes, how would I want to be treated?"

What if the Golden Rule became the gold standard of how you treated others?

The Golden Rule Guardrails

On most curvy highways, there are silver guardrails lining the bends in the road. Their purpose is to keep drivers from going off the road or cliff. I have a few suggested guardrails that will help you treat others the way you would like to be treated.

Honor. "Honor one another above yourselves" (Romans 12:10). To treat people with honor is to treat them with dignity and respect. It's placing a high value on them. It's remembering that every person you encounter is made in the image of God (see

Genesis 1:26). They are God's masterpiece (see Ephesians 2:10). They are "fearfully and wonderfully made" (Psalm 139:14). Honor means remembering that the person in front of you is so valuable to Jesus that He died on the cross for them.

In the leadership book *The Servant,* James Hunter tells a fictional story about a man who spent a week learning about servant leadership in a convent. During one of the scenes, a nurse makes an impactful statement on how to honor others. She said:

> One of the mentors in my life was my first charge nurse in Labor and Delivery nearly twenty years ago. She once confided in me that she liked to picture in her mind's eye that every employee was wearing one of those sandwich billboard signs. On the front side, the sign would read "Appreciate me," and on the back side "Make me feel important."[2]

Honesty. "Do not lie to each other" (Colossians 3:9). Honesty is telling the truth to one another, and the opposite of honesty is deception. Honesty is the foundation of healthy relationships.

In the *Leadership Challenge*, authors James Kouzes and Barry Posner share the results of an extensive survey they took. They were trying to discern what people look for in a leader. Consistently, the number one answer has not changed over the years: "Honesty."[3] People want their leaders to be honest.

Honesty is the best leadership policy. It is also the best life policy. Without honesty, there is no trust, and without trust, there is no relationship. It starts with honesty. Are you an honest person?

Posner and Kouzes share a practical way to be honest with others: "DWYSYWD." This means, "Do what you say you will do." Make and keep promises with others. If you say you are going to do something, move heaven and earth to do it. People lose trust in you when your actions don't back up your words.

Don't talk behind people's backs. "Brothers and sisters, do not slander one another. Anyone who speaks against a brother or sister or judges them speaks against the law and judges it" (James 4:11).

If you have lived long enough, you have felt the sting of having your name drug through the mud. Maybe someone posted something nasty about you on social media. Perhaps you overheard that someone was spreading lies about you. It hurts. Recall this pain when you are tempted to slander someone behind their back. Be faithful to those who are not present. If someone starts bad-mouthing another not in the room, walk away. Or say something nice about the absent person. Or ask the slanderer, "Have you spoken to them about this?" I read somewhere that to belittle others is to *be little*.

Encouragement. "Therefore encourage one another and build each other up, just as in fact you are doing" (1 Thessalonians 5:11). Would others consider you an encourager? Do the words you habitually use build others up or tear them down? "The tongue has the power of life and death" (Proverbs 18:21). The words you speak can plant a seed of life or death in another person. Choose your words prayerfully and thoughtfully.

As you journey through your day, remember that most people you encounter are fighting a difficult battle. Their marriage may be hanging on by a string, their family may be divided over politics, or their health may be falling apart. You can bless them by encouraging them. Your words can breathe courage into them and motivate them to keep on keeping on.

At the beginning of our new church, we held services in rented facilities for several years. Setting up and taking down our equipment every Sunday was starting to wear on the faithful few who helped every week. We started to dream of building our own church building. A place we could call home. We had the property; we just needed the funds to build.

Enthusiastically, I asked one of our board members to look at our books to see if we could afford to build. He responded with a dismal report, "We can't afford to build."

When he said those words, I felt the life drain out of me like air being let out of a tire. My shoulders sank.

Wait. He wasn't done talking. He then said something I have never forgotten, "We can't afford to build . . . *but we are in the faith business, aren't we?*"

When he added that last sentence, I could feel my faith rise. I put my shoulders back and reminded myself that all things are possible with God (see Mark 10:27).

By God's grace, our little church was able to build within a few years. I look back on that man's words as pivotal in my faith journey: We are in the faith business, aren't we?

No matter what difficulty you are facing today, I want to remind you that as a follower of Jesus, you are in the faith business. With God, all things are possible (see Matthew 19:26). Don't give up; look up and trust that He can do immeasurably more than you can ask or imagine (see Ephesians 3:20).

Keep Your Compass Close

As you go throughout your day today, ask this question: If I were in their shoes, how would I want to be treated?

BEYOND THE BOOK

Takeaway: Make the Golden Rule the gold standard of how you treat people. Before you act, take out the compass of the Golden Rule and ask, "If I were in their shoes, how would I want to be treated?"

Verse to memorize: "So in everything, do to others what you would have them do to you, for this sums up the Law and the Prophets" (Matthew 7:12)

Questions to consider: Do you treat people with honor, honesty, encouragement? Do you refrain from talking negatively behind people's backs?

Reflections:

Prayer: *Lord, help me make the Golden Rule my compass for treating others. Before I react to others, help me push the pause button and ask, "If I were in their shoes, how would I want to be treated?" By faith, I will let the Golden Rule, not momentary feelings, guide my actions. Amen.*

Application: Imagine some challenging situations you have experienced recently with others. Ask yourself, "If I were in their shoes, how would I want to be treated?" Then, visualize yourself proactively applying the Golden Rule so that you are ready the next time it happens in real time.

CHAPTER TWENTY-EIGHT

The Strategy for Self-Care

Watch your life and doctrine closely. Persevere in them, because if you do, you will save both yourself and your hearers.

1 Timothy 4:16

How did I get so low? What led to my breakdown? How did I end up so empty? I pondered those questions on my sabbatical in the summer of 2002. As I reflected, I came to understand that one of the major contributing factors was my faulty view of self-care.

Self-care is selfish, I erroneously thought. As a result, I worked day and night. When I wasn't working, I felt guilty. *I should be doing something.* There were always people to visit, sermons to write, and emails to respond to. This out-of-control schedule caught up with me that summer.

Everything changed, however, when I asked a simple question: Does the Bible teach that self-care is selfish? Did Jesus teach that self-care is selfish?

No!

"Love your neighbor *as yourself*" (Matthew 22:39, emphasis added). We are to love ourselves. One way you can do this is by taking care of yourself. This is not referring to selfishness but rather self-care. Roy Oswald calls this practice "self-care for the sake of the kingdom. I take care of myself, not only for my sake . . . but also for the sake of others."[1]

A great example of this is riding on an airplane. Before take-off, a flight attendant will grab the mic and give the safety spiel. "If cabin pressure is lost, oxygen masks will drop from above you. Pull the mask toward you, place it over your nose and mouth, and breathe normally. Secure your own mask before helping others."

Why do they instruct us to secure our own mask before helping others? We need oxygen in our own systems to be able to help others. If we are suffocating and gasping for air, we will pass out instead of being able to help others. Self-care is like putting on an air mask so that you can better help others. The healthier you are, the more people you can help.

> Self-care is never a selfish act—it is simply good stewardship of the only gift I have, the gift I was put on earth to offer others. Anytime we can listen to our true self and give it the care it requires, we do so not only for ourselves but for the many others whose lives we touch.[2]

But What I Do Have, I Give You

Walking to the temple to pray, Peter and John encountered a lame man. He had been this way since birth. The man asked them if they could spare some money.

> "Silver or gold I do not have, *but what I do have I give you*. In the name of Jesus Christ of Nazareth, walk." Taking him by the right hand, he helped him up, and instantly the man's feet and ankles became strong.
>
> Acts 3:6–7, emphasis added

Besides teaching about the supernatural power of God to heal, this Scripture passage teaches a crucial spiritual principle: We cannot give away what we don't have. Note the sentence, "What I do have I give you."

You can only give what you have. If you have food, you can give it away. If you don't, you can't. It's the same with your spirit. If your spiritual, emotional, and mental tank is full, you have the ability to bless others. If it's empty, you don't.

What if your new attitude was, "I am filling my cup so that I have an overflow to share with others"?

Here are three other reasons to prioritize filling up your self-care cup:

Jesus modeled it. "But Jesus often withdrew to lonely places and prayed" (Luke 5:16). Jesus was extremely busy during His three years of open ministry. "Large crowds from Galilee, the Decapolis, Jerusalem, Judea and the region across the Jordan followed him" (Matthew 4:25). Yet we see Him proactively carving out time in His busy schedule to commune with His heavenly Father.

He didn't hope for time; He made time!

"Isn't that selfish?" someone asks. "Shouldn't Jesus have been focused on helping others? Comforting the low-spirited? Healing the sick?"

No! Jesus prioritized time with the Father because he knew, "The Son can do nothing by himself; he can do only what he sees his Father doing" (John 5:19).

Walking on eggshells? Have you ever considered what it is like to live with you? Work with you? Do others walk on eggshells around you? Are you continually tired and irritable? Someone sadly quipped, "Home is where you go when you are sick of being nice to people." Does that describe your presence at home?"

If so, there is a good chance you have failed to put the air mask on yourself. Empty people are often irritable, angry, and short-fused. They are like Grumpy in *Snow White and the Seven Dwarfs*—cynical, bad-tempered, and touchy. Do others refer to you as grumpy? If so, it could stem from a lack of self-care.

Temptation 101. Phillips Brooks said about temptation:

Some day in the years to come, [you will be] wrestling with the great temptation or trembling . . . under the great sorrow of your life.

. . . But the real struggle is not *then*, but *now*—here, on this quiet day and in these quiet weeks. *Now* it is being decided whether, in the day of your supreme sorrow or temptation, you shall miserably fail or gloriously conquer.[3]

Today is the day to prepare for tomorrow's temptations. One of the best ways to do that is to keep our emotional and spiritual buckets full. Why? We are most susceptible to temptation when we are running on fumes.

Specifically, we need to be on guard during four seasons. One way to reference this is through the acronym HALT:[4]

- *Hungry.* In addition to being hungry for food, you can be hungry for love, attention, or meaning. When you are not getting affection at home, you are more susceptible to the flirtations of a coworker.
- *Angry.* I once read that anger is one letter removed from danger. Why? Uncontrolled anger can cause us to say nasty words and engage in cruel actions.
- *Lonely.* One of Satan's favorite tactics is to isolate us. He can tempt us to fill that loneliness hole with forbidden fruit.
- *Tired.* "Fatigue makes cowards of us all."[5]

Driven or Called?

By nature, I am an ambitious person. In many ways, that ambition has really blessed me—achieving a lot and gaining esteem in the eyes of others. In other ways, it has been a curse. In the early days, for example, my ambition led me to focus excessively on outer fruit—the growth and numbers of the ministry. This laser-like focus on numbers blinded me to the state of my soul.

Being at a church for over twenty-five years means going through different seasons. During one series of explosive growth, I felt miserable. I was living out what David Seamands in *Healing Grace* called the superself,[6] which means looking full and healthy on the outside but being empty on the inside. I didn't understand what was happening, so I asked the Lord for guidance. I sensed Him tell me, *You are so focused on outer fruit; what about inner fruit?* After that revelation, I made a promise to myself. From that day forward, I wanted to balance outer fruit—growth of the ministry—with inner fruit—displaying love, joy, peace, etc. The book *Ordering Your Private World* by Gordon MacDonald helped me do that. In it, he talks about the difference between a driven person and a called person.

A driven person is

- most often gratified only by accomplishment;
- preoccupied with the symbols of accomplishment;
- usually caught in the uncontrolled pursuit of expansion;
- tends to have a limited regard for integrity;
- is not likely to bother with the honing of people skills;
- tends to be highly competitive;
- often possesses a volcanic force of anger;
- is usually abnormally busy, averse to play, and avoids spiritual worship.[7]

For the most part, this list fit me back in 2002. Over the past twenty-four years, I have sought to move from being a driven leader to a called one. According to MacDonald, John the Baptist is a good example of a called leader.

> To this John replied, "A person can receive only what is given them from heaven. You yourselves can testify that I said, 'I am not the Messiah but am sent ahead of him.' The bride belongs to the bridegroom. The friend who attends the bridegroom waits and listens for him, and is full of joy when he hears the bridegroom's voice. That joy is mine, and it is now complete. He must become greater; I must become less."
>
> John 3:27–30

A called leader

- appreciates grace, recognizing that everything they have comes from the gracious hand of God;
- avoids the messiah complex, understanding that they cannot fix others—that is Jesus' job; they live according to the Stephen Ministry slogan, "God is the cure giver; I am the caregiver";
- anticipates hearing the voice of the bridegroom, seeking to hear His voice above all others;
- asks God for more humility, praying, "He must increase; I must become less."[8]

Are you a driven person or a called one? Are you following the Good Shepherd's voice or a driven taskmaster?

BEYOND THE BOOK

Takeaway: Practice sacrificial self-care, which believes, "I am taking care of myself for you." Put the oxygen mask on yourself before helping others.

Verse to memorize: "The LORD is my shepherd, I lack nothing. He makes me lie down in green pastures, he leads me beside quiet waters, he refreshes my soul. He guides me along the right paths for his name's sake" (Psalm 23:1–3).

Questions to consider: Am I driven or called? If so, where did this come from?

Reflections: _____

_____

_____

_____

_____

_____

Prayer: *Lord, thank You for modeling self-care to me. Please help me to take time to care for myself so that I can care for others. Help me move from being driven to being called. By faith, I chose to make You my Good Shepherd and listen to Your voice as You lead me into green pastures and quiet waters. May You increase and I decrease. Amen.*

Application: Develop a self-care plan that includes all four keys: mental, physical, spiritual, and relational.

Spiritual	Mental
Physical	Relational

The Checklist of Care

Do not merely listen to the word. . . . Do what it says.

James 1:22

The Gains of the Gathering Years

Develop a holistic view of your mental well-being:

- Spiritual—you are the steward of your spirit.
- Mental—you are the manager of your mind.
- Physical—you are the strategist of your strength.
- Relational—you are the nurturer of your networks.

The Danger of Denial

Can you relate to the symptoms of David's depression?

Y or N: Crying and sadness

Y or N: Physical ailments

Y or N: Loss of purpose

Y or N: Dietary changes

Y or N: Loneliness
Y or N: Sleep disturbances

Set up an appointment with your primary care physician if you are wrestling with these symptoms.

The Victory of Vulnerability

You may feel alone. You are not.

Avoid the "illness/isolation" cycle. If you feel like isolating, acknowledge it and reach out to others in faith.

Avoid the "victorious Christian" paradigm: *If I have problems, it means I don't have enough faith.*

Find a trusted few with whom you can be vulnerable. Victory comes from vulnerability.

The Stigma of Shame

Avoid the stigma of mental illness. We are all broken, just in different ways.

Are you listening to the voice of shame or guilt? Guilt says you did wrong. Shame says you are wrong.

Grace says you can do nothing to make God love you more or less. He loves you based on His loving nature, not your behavior.

The Cost of Control

Are you believing the illusion of control? Are you acting as though you have control over things that you don't?

Ask yourself: Is it a fact of life—something you have no control over, or a problem—something you can do something about? Accept the facts of life and focus on solving your problems with God's help.

The Impact of Identity

Watch out for the Identity Traps.

    T or F: I am how I look.

    T or F: I am who my bank account says I am.

    T or F: I am what I achieve.

    T or F: I am who others say I am.

    T or F: I am what I have done in the past.

    T or F: I am my illness.

    T or F: I am who I AM says that I am.

The Healing of Hope

Don't act on suicidal thoughts. Get help.

How full is your hope bucket? Empty? Halfway? Full?

Remember God's faithfulness in the past. The same God who got you through the storms of yesterday will get you through your present ones.

Anticipate a breakthrough. Trust God.

Be persistent. Don't give up. Do the next right thing.

The Value of Values

Is your focus on *doing* for Jesus or *being* with Him?

What are your top five to seven core values?

Do a values audit.

Live in the *and*. Acknowledge your feelings *and* chose to live according to your values.

Make value-based decisions. Ask yourself what you can do today that will lead you toward your core values.

The Call of Compassion

Try the Compassion Cure. Ask yourself every day, "Who can I help today?"

Compassion is good for your mental health. In lifting others, you rise.

Practice self-compassion. After acknowledging your feelings, ask, "How can I show empathy and express encouragement to myself?"

Meditate on God's compassion. As you would anticipate a fresh pot of coffee, anticipate God's compassion every morning.

The Gift of Gratitude

God's will for you is to be thankful. Develop an attitude of gratitude.

Ponder the goodness of God (see Psalm 16).

Practice the other side of the coin exercise. List the negative aspects of the situation and then list the positive aspects.

Bookend your day with gratitude. Begin and end the day with gratitude.

The Antidote to Anxiety

Worrying is an expensive habit. Ponder how much it has cost you.

Estimate the validity quotient of your worries. How many times in the past have your worries come true?

Live in day-tight compartments. Live one day at a time.

Live in the focused mode. Try to anchor yourself in the present moment.

Practice: Feel, Ignore, Engage.

The Training of Thoughts

Recall the power of your thoughts. Your thoughts can change your biology.

Take your thoughts captive. Cast the unhealthy thoughts out of your mind.

Be on guard for the seven toxic thoughts:

- Pessimistic forecast
- Undervaluing your resilience in Christ
- Negative assessment
- Brooding over
- All-or-nothing thinking
- Overgeneralization
- Personalizing

The Function of Feelings

Name your emotions. Say, "I am feeling _____."

Don't worship your feelings or demonize them. Feel them. Consider them to be like the dashboard lights on your car. They are trying to communicate something to you.

Examine your self-talk. How you talk to yourself determines your feelings. Feel your feelings.

Pray a prayer of lament.

The Joy of Journaling

Practice paper therapy. Write the thoughts and feelings swirling in your head and heart on paper.

Document your journey with God.

Be aware of your explanatory style. How do you explain things to yourself? Are those explanations accurate?

Experiment with journal exercises:

- ABCDE
- What's bothering me
- The morning download
- Scripture writing

The Test of the Truth

Look for the two ingredients of truth: Is it reliable? Is it biblical?

Practice the three steps for overcoming deception:
- Locate the lies.
- Replace the lies with the truth.
- Argue against lies.

Remember the three weapons against Satan:
- The name of Jesus (see Philippians 2:10)
- The blood of Jesus (see Revelation 12:11)
- The Word of God (see Ephesians 6:11)

The Cause for Contentment

You are on a journey to be yourself. Don't try to be a second-class version of someone else. Be a first-class version of yourself.

What gifts has God placed in your box?

Contented Christians use their gifts for God's glory.

Avoid the weakness obsession.

By faith, declare: "When I am weak, Jesus is strong!"

The Effects of Exercise

Motion affects emotions.

Exercising will give you more energy to live for Christ.

Recall the benefits of exercise:

- It sharpens your brain.
- It increases your energy.
- It shows gratitude to God, and it can help you serve God better and longer.
- It helps you cope with depression and anxiety.
- It helps you sleep better.

The Nature of Nutrition

Food affects mood.

Eat food that is whole, fresh, and unprocessed.

Eat food for nutritional reasons. Before you eat, ask yourself why you are eating this.

Stop eating when you are 80 percent full.

Eat with an eye for the future. What will the effect of this food choice be in ten minutes, ten months, and ten years?

The Habit of Hydration

Dehydration is dangerous for your brain.

A hydrated brain is a happy brain.

Practice Blue Mind Theory.

Don't wait until you feel thirsty to drink water. Drink water proactively, not reactively.

Be aware of the symptoms of dehydration:

- Depression
- Afternoon fatigue
- Sleep issues
- Inability to focus
- Lack of mental clarity, sometimes called brain fog
- Dark urine

The Duty of Delight

Work hard and play hard.

Laugh like Jesus.

Develop some delightful diversions.

Let children mentor. Learn how to laugh and have fun from them.

Develop and use a life-giving list.

Leverage time off and vacation. Rest makes you your best.

Have a weekly Sabbath. On your Sabbath ask, "How can I pray and play today?"

The Myths About Medication

Mental illness can stem from a biological source. We are multifaceted beings—body, soul, and spirit.

Be open to Jesus healing you naturally or supernaturally. He may choose to heal you through a miracle or medicine.

Take your prescribed medication on a consistent basis. Don't deviate from your medicine without consulting your doctor.

The Spirituality of Sleep

Do a sleep audit.

Make a sleep routine.

Recall the benefits of good sleep:
- It regulates the release of essential hormones.
- It slows the aging process.
- It boosts your immune system.
- It improves brain function.
- It reduces cortisol levels.

Process your stress before bed.

Take naps.

Be humble enough to admit you need sleep.

The Call of Connection

Loneliness and isolation increase your likeliness of death and disease.

Our society programs us for loneliness.

To be healthy and whole, you need others.

Remember the lesson of coals. Just as coals warm each other, believers do the same as they fellowship together.

Find your Brock and Bennet. Initiate ways to develop deeper connections with others.

The Blessings of Boundaries

Boundaries define what is within your yard of responsibility.

Focus on self-control, not the control of others.

Develop the attitude of boundaries:

- I am one-hundred-percent responsible for my attitude, actions, and lifestyle.
- I am not responsible for other people's actions and lifestyles.
- I can influence others but not control them.

Respect other people's boundaries.

The Force of Family

There are no perfect families in the Bible. Even Jesus' family had issues.

Be aware of how your childhood shaped you.

Become a transitional person. Determine not to pass down to the next generation the unhealthy patterns you were given. Align your behavior to your new family, the family of God.

The Elements of Empathy

Empathize and then explain. Before you share your viewpoint, take time to understand the other person's view.

Listen and acknowledge the feelings behind a person's message.

Practice the three R's:

- Restate content.
- Reflect feeling.
- Render empathy.

Recall the advice from the FBI hostage negotiator:

- Actively listen.
- Show empathy.
- Build trust.
- Foster collaboration.

The Freedom of Forgiveness

Forgiveness is sending away the hurt to God.

Forgive because Jesus has forgiven you.

$E + R = O$

Don't ask what is wrong with them. Ask what happened to them. Have you heard their story?

Pray for those who have hurt you. "It hurt. It mattered. But I forgive you and wish you well."

Love your enemies.

The Guidance of the Golden Rule

Make the Golden Rule your relational compass. Continually ask yourself how you would want to be treated if you were in another person's shoes.

Recall the four guardrails:

Honor: "They are God's masterpiece."

Honesty: DWYSYWD. Do what you say you will do.

Don't slander others behind their backs.

Encourage others: "I believe in you."

The Strategy for Self-Care

Practice "sacrificial self-care." Have the attitude, "I am taking care of me for you."

Ask yourself, "What's it like to live with me?" Like Grumpy? Do others walk on eggshells?

Jesus modeled self-care. He spent time with the Father.

Am I a driven or called leader? Ask, how can I make strides to move from "driven" to "called?"

Be on guard during seasons of HALT:

Hungry?

Angry?

Lonely?

Tired?

Work Your Program

Thank you for taking this journey with me. My hope is that you won't simply place this book on a shelf and move on, but that you'll return to it—rereading, reflecting, and practicing its lessons—until they begin to reshape you from the inside out.

One of the key attitudes I've developed is this: I need to work my program. Just as someone in recovery commits to meetings, a sponsor, and daily readings, I've come to see that I need to consistently live out these four principles—spiritual, mental, physical, and relational—if I want to grow in health and wholeness.

May God help you stay close to Jesus and faithfully work your program, one day at a time.

Notes

Introduction The Gains of the Gathering Years

1. Nancy Koehn, *Forged in Crisis: The Power of Courageous Leadership in Turbulent Times* (Simon and Schuster, 2017), 6.
2. Roy Oswald, *Clergy Self-Care: Finding a Balance for Effective Ministry* (Alban Institute, 1998), 10.

Chapter 1 The Danger of Denial

1. Leighton Ford, *The Attentive Life: Discerning God's Presence in All Things* (IVP Books, 2008), 143.
2. Craig Sawchuk, "Depression (Major Depressive Disorder)," Mayo Clinic, October 14, 2022, https://www.mayoclinic.org/diseases-conditions/depression /symptoms-causes/syc-20356007.
3. Keith Kramlinger, ed., *Mayo Clinic on Depression: Answers to Help You Understand, Recognize and Manage Depression* (Mayo Clinic, 2001), 3.
4. Tim Clinton, *The Soul Care Bible: Experiencing and Sharing Hope God's Way* (Thomas Nelson, 2001), 780.
5. John R. O'Neil, *The Paradox of Success: When Winning at Work Means Losing at Life* (G. P. Putnam's Sons, 1993), 155.
6. Quoted in Amy Carmichael, *Though the Mountains Shake* (Loizeaux Brothers, 1946), 12.

Chapter 2 The Victory of Vulnerability

1. John Mark Comer, *The Ruthless Elimination of Hurry: How to Stay Emotionally Healthy and Spiritually Alive in the Chaos of the Modern World* (WaterBrook, 2019), 134.
2. Amy Simpson, *Troubled Minds: Mental Illness and the Church's Mission* (IVP Books, 2013), 16.
3. Simpson, *Troubled Minds*, 104–105.

4. Edward Gilbreath, "Level Ground at the Cross," *Christianity Today*, April 2018, https://www.christianitytoday.com/2018/02/level-ground-at-cross/.

5. Philip Yancey, *What's So Amazing About Grace?* (Zondervan, 1997), 276.

6. Joan Borysenko, "The Blessings of Imperfection," *Prevention*, May 2004, repr., https://joanborysenko.com/mind-body-balance/maintaining-a-healthy-balance/the-blessings-of-imperfection/.

Chapter 3 The Stigma of Shame

1. Chris Hodges, *Out of the Cave: Stepping into the Light When Depression Darkens What You See* (Nelson Books, 2021), 37.

2. Department of Health and Human Services, *Mental Health: A Report of the Surgeon General* (National Institute of Mental Health, 1999), 3, https://profiles.nlm.nih.gov/spotlight/nn/catalog/nlm:nlmuid-101584932X120-doc.

3. Jeff VanVonderen, *Tired of Trying to Measure Up: Getting Free from the Demands, Expectations, and Intimidation of Well-Meaning People* (Bethany House, 1989), 19.

4. Lewis B. Smedes, *Shame and Grace: Healing the Shame We Don't Deserve* (HarperOne, 2009), 67.

5. Yancey, *What's So Amazing About Grace?*, 70.

6. Timothy Keller, *Preaching: Communicating Faith in an Age of Skepticism* (Viking, 2015), 52.

Chapter 4 The Cost of Control

1. Ellen Langer, "The Illusion of Control," *Journal of Personality and Social Psychology* 32, no. 2 (1975), https://psycnet.apa.org/doiLanding?doi=10.1037%2F0022-3514.32.2.311.

2. Hodges, *Out of the Cave*, 153.

3. Reinhold Niebuhr, "The Original Serenity Prayer," Proactive 12 Steps, accessed July 25, 2025, https://proactive12steps.com/serenity-prayer/.

4. Henry Blackaby and Claude King, *Experiencing God: How to Live the Full Adventure of Knowing and Doing the Will of God* (Broadman & Holman, 1994), 25.

5. Ronald Klug, *How to Keep a Spiritual Journal: A Guide to Journal Keeping for Inner Growth and Personal Discovery* (Augsburg, 1993), 13.

6. Andrew Newberg and Mark Robert Waldman, *How God Changes Your Brain: Breakthrough Findings from a Leading Neuroscientist* (Ballantine Books, 2009), 149.

7. Newberg and Waldman, *How God Changes Your Brain*, 48.

Chapter 5 The Impact of Identity

1. William Backus and Marie Chapian, *Telling Yourself the Truth: Find Your Way Out of Depression, Anxiety, Fear, Anger, and Other Common Problems by Applying the Principles of Misbelief Therapy* (Bethany House, 2014), 41.

2. Alex Kendrick and Stephen Kendrick, *Defined: Who God Says You Are* (B&H, 2019), 11.

3. Kendrick and Kendrick, *Defined*, 109.

4. George H. Mead, *Mind, Self and Society: From the Standpoint of a Social Behaviorist* (University of Chicago Press, 1934), 90.

5. Leighton Ford, *Transforming Leadership: Jesus' Way of Creating Vision, Shaping Values & Empowering Change* (IVP Books, 2010), 92.

6. Yancey, *What's So Amazing About Grace?*, 68–69.

7. Blackaby and King, *Experiencing God*, 53.

Chapter 6 The Healing of Hope

1. Kramlinger, *Mayo Clinic on Depression*, 16.

2. Adapted from an old Taoist story, told in Wayne Muller, *Sabbath: Finding Rest, Renewal, and Delight in Our Busy Lives* (Bantam Books, 1999), 187.

3. Ted Engstrom and Paul Cedar, *Compassionate Leadership: Rediscovering Jesus' Radical Leadership Style* (Baker Books, 2011), 44.

4. Anne Lamott, *Bird by Bird: Some Instructions on Writing and Life*, 25th anniv. ed. (Anchor Books, 2019), xxiv.

5. H. Dale Burke, *Less Is More Leadership: 8 Secrets to How to Lead and Still Have a Life* (Harvest House, 2004), 222–223.

Chapter 7 The Value of Values

1. Patrick Klingaman, *Finding Rest When the Work Is Never Done* (David C. Cook, 2002), 98.

2. Paul Sangster, *Doctor Sangster* (Epworth Press, 1962), 342.

3. Comer, *The Ruthless Elimination of Hurry*, 20.

4. David Vaughan, *Jonathan Edwards* (Bethany House, 2000), 23.

5. Richard Swenson, *In Search of Balance: Keys to a Stable Life* (Tyndale, 2014), 65–66.

6. Swenson, *In Search of Balance*, 85.

7. Newberg and Waldman, *How God Changes Your Brain*, 20.

Chapter 8 The Call of Compassion

1. Mother Teresa, "Mother Teresa at the National Prayer Breakfast," EWTN, February 3, 1994, https://www.ewtn.com/catholicism/library/mother-teresa-at-the-national-prayer-breakfast-2714.

2. Carol Zaleski, "The Dark Night of Mother Teresa," *First Things*, May 1, 2003, https://firstthings.com/the-dark-night-of-mother-teresa/.

3. Quoted in Andrew Farley, *The Naked Gospel: The Truth You May Never Hear in Church* (Zondervan, 2009), 35.

4. "What Does the Bible Say About Compassion?," Got Questions Ministries, page last updated November 13, 2023, https://www.gotquestions.org/Bible-compassion.html.

5. Engstrom and Cedar, *Compassionate Leadership*, 45.

6. Amit Sood, *The Mayo Clinic Guide to Stress-Free Living* (Balance, 2013), 94.

7. John Keble, *Letters of Spiritual Counsel and Guidance*, 2nd ed. (Oxford and London, 1870), 6.

Chapter 9 The Gift of Gratitude

1. Og Mandino, *Og Mandino's University of Success* (Bantam, 2011), 18–19.

2. Dale Carnegie, *How to Stop Worrying and Start Living* (Windmill Press, 1949), 131.

3. Billy Graham, "What Billy Graham Had to Say About His Homegoing," Billy Graham Library, February 17, 2020, https://billygrahamlibrary.org/blog-what-billy-graham-had-to-say-about-his-homegoing/.

Chapter 10 The Antidote to Anxiety

1. Paul Daugherty, *Mind Games: Winning the Battle for Your Mental and Emotional Health* (Faith Words, 2024), 89.

2. Charles Stone, *People-Pleasing Pastors: Avoiding the Pitfalls of Approval-Motivated Leadership* (IVP, 2014), 47.

3. *Field of Dreams*, Phil Alden Robinson, Universal Pictures, 1989, 38:53.

4. Seth Gilihan, "How Often Do Your Worries Actually Come True?," *Psychology Today*, July 19, 2019, https://www.psychologytoday.com/us/blog/think-act-be/201907/how-often-do-your-worries-actually-come-true.

5. William Osler, quoted in Carnegie, *How to Stop Worrying*, 2.

6. Klingaman, *Finding Rest*, 51.

7. Sood, *Stress-Free Living*, 3–4.

8. Henry Cloud, *Boundaries.me*, podcast, episode 333, "The Dr. Cloud Show Live—Special Edition: Spotlight on Anxiety," March 28, 2022, https://boundaries.libsyn.com/episode-333-the-dr-cloud-show-live-spotlight-on-anxiety.

9. Steve Cuss, *Managing Leadership Anxiety: Yours and Theirs* (Thomas Nelson, 2019), 17.

10. Matthew McKay, Patrick Fanning, and Patricia Zurita Ona, *Mind and Emotions: A Universal Treatment for Emotional Disorders* (New Harbinger Publications, 2011), 75.

Chapter 11 The Training of Thoughts

1. Backus and Chapian, *Telling Yourself the Truth*, 26.

2. Old Sarum Primer, "God Be in My Head," A Collection of Prayers, June 22, 2016, https://acollectionofprayers.com/2016/06/22/god-be-in-my-head/.

3. Stone, *People-Pleasing Pastors*, 163.

4. McKay, Fanning, and Ona, *Mind and Emotions*, 87.

Chapter 12 The Function of Feelings

1. This retreat was conducted by a ministry of Focus on the Family called Hope Restored. For more information, visit https://hoperestored.focusonthefamily.com/marriage-intensives-save-your-marriage/.

2. Mark Vroegop, *Dark Clouds, Deep Mercy: Discovering the Grace of Lament* (Crossway, 2019), 26.

3. Gary Neal Hansen, *Kneeling with Giants: Learning to Pray with History's Best Teachers* (IVP, 2012), 78.

4. Andriy Nurzhynskyy, "Basic Emotions: A Guide to Understanding the 6 Core Human Feelings," Psychology, accessed July 25, 2025, https://psychology.tips/basic-emotions/.

5. Gary Smalley, *The DNA of Relationships: Discover How You Are Designed for Satisfying Relationships* (Tyndale, 2013), 93.

6. Rick Warren, *The Purpose-Driven Life: What on Earth Am I Here For?* (Zondervan, 2002), 64.

7. McKay, Fanning, and Ona, *Mind and Emotions*, 12.

8. Brian Tracy, "95% of your emotions," Facebook, November 14, 2017, https://www.facebook.com/BrianTracyPage/posts/95-of-your-emotions-are-determined-by-the-way-you-talk-to-yourself-youd-be-surpr/10155249166853460/.

9. Martin Seligman, *Learned Optimism: How to Change Your Mind and Your Life* (Vintage, 2006), 238.

10. Vroegop, *Dark Clouds, Deep Mercy*, 29.

Chapter 13 The Joy of Journaling

1. John Thornburry, *David Brainerd: Pioneer Missionary to the American Indians* (Evangelical Press, 1996), 15.

2. John Piper, "His Suffering Sparked a Movement," Desiring God, April 20, 2018, https://www.desiringgod.org/articles/his-suffering-sparked-a-movement.

3. John Piper, *The Hidden Smile of God: The Fruit of Affliction in the Lives of John Bunyan, William Cowper, and David Brainerd* (Crossway Books, 2001), 135.

4. Anne Frank, *The Diary of a Young Girl* (Bantam, 1993), 5.

5. Klug, *How to Keep a Spiritual Journal*, 11.

6. Quoted in Rick Warren, *The Purpose-Driven Church: Growth Without Compromising Your Message & Mission* (Zondervan, 1995), 99.

7. Seligman, *Learned Optimism*, 40.

8. Michael Bungay Stanier, *The Coaching Habit: Say Less, Ask More & Change the Way You Lead Forever* (Box of Crayons Press, 2016), 48.

9. Daniel Kahneman, *Thinking Fast and Slow* (Farrar, Straus, and Giroux, 2011).

10. Peter Skoog, Peter Greer, and Cameron Doolittle, *Lead with Prayer: The Spiritual Habits of World-Changing Leaders* (Faith Words, 2024), 24.

Chapter 14 The Test of the Truth

1. G. W. Knight and R. W. Ray, *Layman's Bible Dictionary* (Barbour, 2012), 330.

2. Backus and Chapian, *Telling Yourself the Truth*, 13.

3. Becky Meyerson, "The Volcano: A Tool for Managing My Thoughts," accessed July 25, 2025, https://www.beckymeyerson.com/volcano.

4. J. Robert Clinton, *The Making of a Leader: Recognizing the Lessons and Stages of Leadership Development* (NavPress, 1988), 113.

5. Matthew Stanford, *Grace for the Afflicted: A Clinical and Biblical Perspective on Mental Illness* (IVP Books, 2008), 35.

6. Archibald Hart, *Mastering Pastoral Counseling* (Thomas Nelson, 1991), 59.

Chapter 15 The Cause for Contentment

1. Tom Rath and Barry Conchie, *Strengths Based Leadership: Great Leaders, Teams, and Why People Follow* (Gallup Press, 2008), 13.
2. Blackaby and King, *Experiencing God*, 29.
3. Gene Edwards, *A Tale of Three Kings: A Study in Brokenness* (Tyndale, 1992), 28.
4. Christian Schwarz, *Natural Church Development* (Church Smart Resources, 2003), 24.
5. Howard Gardner, *Frames of Mind: The Theory of Multiple Intelligences* (Basic Books, 2011).
6. Blackaby and King, *Experiencing God*, 20.
7. *Chariots of Fire*, Hugh Hudsen, Warner Bros. Pictures, 1981, 59:12.

Chapter 16 The Effects of Exercise

1. John Ratey and Eric Hagerman, *Spark: The Revolutionary New Science of Exercise and the Brain* (Little, Brown, 2008), 5.
2. Ratey and Hagerman, *Spark*, 11.
3. Steven Covey, *The 7 Habits of Highly Effective People: Powerful Lessons in Personal Change* (Simon and Schuster, 1989), 289.
4. Newberg and Waldman, *How God Changes Your Brain*, 161.
5. Skoog, Greer, and Doolittle, *Lead with Prayer*, 19.
6. Roger Reynolds, "Just As I Am Wellness Seminar," held at the Cooper Institute for Aerobics Research, Dallas, Texas, October 15, 1998, cited by Deborah Newman, *Loving Your Body: Embracing Your True Beauty in Christ* (Tyndale, 2002), 78.

Chapter 17 The Nature of Nutrition

1. Richard Smith, "Let Food Be Thy Medicine," *British Medical Journal* 328, no. 7443 (January 24, 2004), https://pmc.ncbi.nlm.nih.gov/articles/PMC318470/.
2. Devon Frye, "The Foods We Eat Do Affect Our Mental Health. Here's the Proof," *Psychology Today*, January 24, 2020, https://www.psychologytoday.com/us/blog/evidence-based-living/202001/the-foods-we-eat-do-affect-our-mental-health-heres-the-proof.
3. Rick Warren, *The Daniel Plan* (Zondervan, 2013), 38.
4. Warren, *Daniel Plan*, 77.
5. Jordan Rubin, *The Maker's Diet: The 40-Day Health Experience That Will Change Your Life Forever* (Destiny Image, 2013), 32.
6. Steve and Mary Farrar, *Overcoming Overload: 7 Ways to Find Rest in Your Chaotic Work* (PRH Christian Publishing, 2004), 95.
7. Dan Buettner, "Hara Hachi Bu: Enjoy Food and Lose Weight With This Simple Japanese Phrase," Blue Zones, updated December 2018, https://www.bluezones.com/2017/12/hara-hachi-bu-enjoy-food-and-lose-weight-with-this-simple-phrase/.
8. Deborah Newman, *Loving Your Body: Embracing Your True Beauty in Christ* (Tyndale, 2002), 79.

Chapter 18 The Habit of Hydration

1. Don Colbert, *Seven Pillars of Health* (Siloam, 2006), 5.

2. Imran Fayaz, "How Dehydration Affects Your Brain," Fayaz Neurosurgery, accessed July 25, 2025, https://fayazneurosurgery.com/how-dehydration-affects -your-brain/.

3. Taylor Leamey, "Here's Why Drinking Water Is the Key to Good Mental Health," CNET, February 1, 2023, https://www.cnet.com/health/mental/heres -why-drinking-water-is-the-key-to-good-mental-health/.

4. Fayaz, "How Dehydration Affects Your Brain."

5. Tom Graney, "The Power of Water," New Life Ranch, November 2, 2021, https://newliferanch.com/blog/the-power-of-water/.

6. SaVanna Shoemaker, "12 Simple Ways to Drink More Water," Healthline, February 10, 2023, https://www.healthline.com/nutrition/how-to-drink-more-water.

7. Wallace Nichols, "What Is Blue Mind theory?" August 22, 2022, https:// www.wallacejnichols.org/126/1835/what-is-blue-mind-theory.html.

Chapter 19 The Duty of Delight

1. Elton Trueblood, *The Humor of Christ* (Harper & Row, 1964).

2. Randy Alcorn, "Do We Miss the Humor of Christ When We Read the Gospels?," Eternal Perspective Ministries, August 5, 2016, https://www.epm.org /resources/2016/Aug/5/humor-christ-gospels/.

3. Trueblood, *Humor of Christ*, 10.

4. Randy Alcorn, *60 Days of Happiness: Discover God's Promise of Relentless Joy* (Tyndale, 2017), 14.

5. "Worship Like You Mean It: Interview with Sally Morgenthaler and Robert Webber," *YouthWorker Journal*, July 1999, https://www.youthworker.com/ worship-like-you-mean-it-interview-with-sally-morgenthaler-and-robert-webber/.

6. O'Neil, *The Paradox of Success*, 167.

7. Ford, *Transforming Leadership*, 92.

8. Klingaman, *Finding Rest*, 103.

9. Richard Exley, *The Rhythm of Life: Putting Life's Priorities in Perspective* (Honor, 1987), 107.

10. Oswald, *Clergy Self-Care*, 132.

Chapter 20 The Myths About Medication

1. Wayne Cordeiro, *Leading on Empty: Refilling Your Tank and Renewing Your Passion* (Bethany House, 2010), 55.

2. "Why Did Jesus Spit for Some of His Miracles?," Got Questions Ministries, page last updated January 4, 2022, https://www.gotquestions.org/Jesus-spit.html.

Chapter 21 The Spirituality of Sleep

1. Jean M. Twenge, "What Makes Teens Happier," *Psychology Today*, August 31, 2018, https://www.psychologytoday.com/us/blog/our-changing-culture/201808 /what-makes-teens-happier.

2. Newberg and Waldman, *How God Changes Your Brain*, 150.

3. Darren Rovell, "Famed 'Be Like Mike' Gatorade Ad Debuted 25 Years Ago," ESPN, August 8, 2016, https://www.espn.com/nba/story/_/id/17246999/michael-jordan-famous-mike-gatorade-commercial-debuted-25-years-ago-monday.

4. John Piper, *Desiring God: Meditations of a Christian Hedonist* (Multnomah Press, 2003), 360.

5. Warren Wiersbe, *Walking with the Giants: A Minister's Guide to Good Reading and Great Preaching* (Baker Book House, 1976), 158.

6. Old Celtic prayer, as quoted by George Hunter III, *The Celtic Way of Evangelism: How Christianity Can Reach the West . . . Again* (Abingdon Press, 2010), 83.

Chapter 22 The Call of Connection

1. Dean Ornish, *Love and Survival: 8 Pathways to Intimacy and Health* (HarperCollins, 1998), 13, 29.

2. Tom Rath and Don Clinton, *How Full Is Your Bucket?* (Gallup Press, 2004), 96.

3. John Burke, *No Perfect People Allowed: Creating a Come-As-You-Are Culture in the Church* (Zondervan, 2005), 270.

4. Sue Johnson, *Created for Connection: The "Hold Me Tight" Guide for Christian Couples* (Little, Brown, 2016), 22.

5. Julian Stratenschulte, "Herd the News? Wild Boar Piglet Adopted by German Cows," *HuffPost*, September 29, 2022, https://www.huffpost.com/entry/german-cows-adopt-boar-piglet_n_633602d1e4b0e376dbf51fc3.

6. Richard Foster, *Celebration of Discipline: The Path to Spiritual Growth* (Harper One, 1988), 172.

Chapter 23 The Blessings of Boundaries

1. Henry Cloud, *Changes That Heal: Four Practical Steps to a Happier, Healthier You* Zondervan, 1996), 92.

2. Niebuhr, "The Original Serenity Prayer."

3. Les Carter, *When Pleasing You Is Killing Me: A Workbook* (B&H Books, 2007), 7.

4. Frederick Buechner, "Marriage," June 20, 2016, https://www.frederickbuechner.com/quote-of-the-day/2016/6/20/marriage.

5. Henry Cloud and John Townsend, *Boundaries: When to Say Yes, When to Say No to Take Control of Your Life* (Zondervan, 2002), 173.

6. Andy Crouch, *The Tech-Wise Family: Everyday Steps for Putting Technology in Its Proper Place* (Baker Books, 2017), 98.

7. Thomas à Kempis, *The Imitation of Christ* (Elliot Stock, Paternoster Row, 1897), 72.

8. Smalley, *DNA of Relationships*, 58.

9. Alice Gray, *Stories for the Heart: Over 100 Stories to Encourage Your Soul* (PRH Christian Publishing,1996), 65.

Chapter 24 The Force of Family

1. Neil S. Wilson, *Life Application Study Bible*, Large Print (Zondervan and Tyndale, 2007), 617.

2. Peter Scazzero, *Emotionally Healthy Spirituality: Unleash a Revolution in Your Life in Christ* (Zondervan, 2006), 95.

3. Kramlinger, *Mayo Clinic on Depression*, 17.

4. Kramlinger, *Mayo Clinic on Depression*, 2.

5. Crouch, *Tech-Wise Family*, 60.

6. Joey Reiman, *Thinking for a Living: Creating Ideas that Revitalize Your Business, Career, and Life* (Long Street Press, 1998), 116.

Chapter 25 The Elements of Empathy

1. Covey, *7 Habits of Highly Effective People*, 239.

2. Smalley, *DNA of Relationships*, 111.

3. Gary Noesner, *Stalling for Time: My Life as an FBI Hostage Negotiator* (Random House, 2010), 12.

Chapter 26 The Freedom of Forgiveness

1. Hansen, *Kneeling with Giants*, 47.

2. Jack Canfield, *The Success Principles: How to Get From Where You Are to Where You Want to Be* (Harper Collins, 2005), 6.

Chapter 27 The Guidance of the Golden Rule

1. Abraham Lincoln, "Lincoln's Unsent Letter to George Meade," American Battlefield Trust, July 14, 1863, https://www.battlefields.org/learn/primary-sources/lincolns-unsent-letter-george-meade.

2. James C. Hunter, *The Servant: A Simple Story About the True Essence of Leadership* (Prima Publishing, 1998), 109.

3. James Kouzes and Barry Posner, *The Leadership Challenge: How to Make Extraordinary Things Happen in Organizations* (Jossy-Bass Inc, 2017), 33.

Chapter 28 The Strategy for Self-Care

1. Oswald, *Clergy Self-Care*, 6.

2. Parker Palmer, *Let Your Life Speak: Listening for the Voice of Vocation* (John Wiley and Sons, 2024), 32.

3. Phillips Brooks, *The More Abundant Life: Lenten Readings* (E. P. Dutton, 1897), 197.

4. David Streem, "HALT: Pay Attention to These Four Stressors on Your Recovery," Cleveland Clinic: Health Essentials, May 24, 2022, https://health.clevelandclinic.org/halt-hungry-angry-lonely-tired.

5. David Chadwick, "Wise Words From Mentors: Fatigue Makes Cowards of Us All," Moments of Hope Church, November 5, 2024, https://www.momentsofhopechurch.org/post/wise-words-from-mentors-fatigue-makes-cowards-of-us-all.

6. David Seamands, *Healing Grace* (Scripture Press, 1988), 99.

7. Gordon MacDonald, *Ordering Your Private World* (Thomas Nelson, 1997), ch. 3.

8. MacDonald, *Ordering Your Private World*, 53.

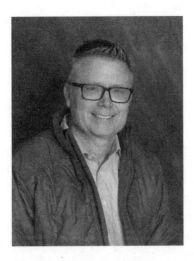

Steve Larson serves as lead pastor of Community Celebration Church in Kasson, Minnesota. God used him and his wife, Tammy, to start the church in 1998. Steve has a down-to-earth teaching style and an authentic, gentle leadership style. His goal is to lead people to an ever-growing relationship with Jesus that balances grace and truth.

He is a passionate writer. His writings have been published in several magazines, and he is a contributing author of *The Church Leader's Answer Book*.

Through years of pastoral ministry, Steve has walked closely with individuals and families navigating mental health challenges. His pastoral care and personal encounters with emotional struggles—both his own and others'—inspired him to write this book with compassion and clarity.

Steve loves learning, traveling, and enjoying family time with Tammy and their two kids, Dalton and Miracle.

CONNECT WITH STEVE:

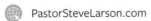 PastorSteveLarson.com

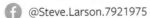 @Steve.Larson.7921975

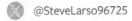 @SteveLarso96725

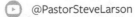 @PastorSteveLarson

Personal Notes

Personal Notes

Personal Notes